Challenges in Cataract Surgery

Wan Soo Kim · Kyeong Hwan Kim

Challenges in Cataract Surgery

Principles and Techniques for Successful Management

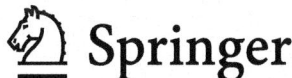

Wan Soo Kim
Busan
South Korea

Kyeong Hwan Kim
Department of Ophthalmology
Inje University College of Medicine
and Haeundae Paik Hospital
Busan
South Korea

ISBN 978-3-662-46091-7   ISBN 978-3-662-46092-4   (eBook)
DOI 10.1007/978-3-662-46092-4

Library of Congress Control Number: 2016955539

Printed on acid-free paper

This Springer imprint is published by Springer Nature
The registered company is Springer-Verlag GmbH Germany
The registered company address is: Heidelberger Platz 3, 14197 Berlin, Germany

To NaHyun, DongHyun and GyooWon
— Wan Soo Kim, MD, PhD

Dedicated to all of my teachers, students, and precious family
— Kim, Kyeong Hwan

Preface and Acknowledgment

I started and became a cataract surgeon when little was known about phaco-surgery, and where courage was more needed than knowledge was. I was lucky enough to meet many teachers who became my friends and friends that became teachers. I would like to thank my dearest friends Dr. Gerd Auffarth, Dr. Abhay Vasavada, Dr. Howard Gimbel, and Dr. David Apple who have influenced my practice as a cataract surgeon more than a couple of decades.

I am lucky to have this book published with my fellow professor, Dr. Kyeong Hwan Kim who has been my colleague for more than a decade. His professional excellence and enthusiasm enabled us to finish this book in fairly short period of time. I also would like to thank my residents (Drs. J. Kim and S. Hwang) for their help during the process of writing.

Tremendous improvement in technology has helped surgeons to overcome challenges in many ways, however, the number of complications following cataract surgeries is not decreasing. I still believe the surgeries are designed and performed by the surgeon, not by sophisticated machines. In this book, I am trying to show you measures and my current surgical techniques to overcome the obstacles we encounter during the course of different cataract surgeries. Please enjoy.

Busan, South Korea   Wan Soo Kim, MD, PhD

Preface

As longevity increases, cataract is becoming an even greater public health issue worldwide. The use of cataract surgery, already one of the most frequently performed surgeries, is consequently increasing still further – a trend reinforced by developments in instrumentation and technology and improvements in access to surgery. However, comorbidities and challenges during surgery are still common.

This book *Challenges in Cataract Surgery* comprises 17 chapters on and around the topic of challenging situations encountered before, during, and after cataract surgery. A wide range of settings are considered, including cataract surgery in patients with intumescent, brunescent, or posterior polar cataract; iris problem; trauma; previous vitrectomy history; uveitis; comorbidities such as glaucoma or corneal diseases; and eyes with unusual axial length. Furthermore, topics such as dislocation of intraocular lens and multifocal intraocular lens are also described.

It is hoped that *Challenges in Cataract Surgery* will be a valuable reference for all residents, fellows, and practicing ophthalmologists who wish to improve their surgical techniques and outcomes, and this first edition will not be the last. And any comments and suggestions from junior and senior readers are welcomed that will help us to make future editions even better.

Busan, South Korea   Kyeong Hwan Kim

Contents

Intumescent Cataract

The intumescent cataract (Fig. 1.1) is not infrequent challenges we encounter in clinical practice. Progression of the cataract to intumescent stage is not predictable, however, systemic conditions such as DM frequently accompanies the intumescent cataract. Because of the distended lens capsule, capsule is thin, stretched zonules are weak or absent, intracapsular pressure is high, there's no red reflex, and they have large rock hard lens nucleus inside. Intumescent cataract,with its distended and disintegrated lens capsule, could develop phacolytic glaucoma (obstruction of the trabecular flow by macrophages scavenged the lens protein released though the loose lens capsule) or phacoanalylaxis (severe inflammation caused by released protein).

Preoperative Considerations

In cases with intumescent cataract, presence of unknown systemic disease or trauma (accidental or surgical) should be asked. As the visual outcome could be undetermined before the surgery, discussion with the patient is necessary to talk about possible complications and the possibility of poor visual outcomes.

AC shallows with the progression of intumescence. If anterior chamber is too shallow, generalized zonular weakening should be anticipated. In intumescent and mature cataract, capsular plaques develop as the capsule degenerates. Some capsules are removed with capsular forceps or polishing needle. As these plaques interfere with creation of intact capsulorhexis (anterior and posterior), capsular scissors of various kinds can be utilized to cut across the plaques (Fig. 1.2).

Evaluation of the visual potential is made by history taking, and B-scan Ultrasound, VEP, Colored light projection and entoptic imagery, however, these tests do not provide accurate prognosis of visual potential, but helps to determine the advantage of cataract surgeries being planned, when the past ocular histories of the patient are not clear.

Phacolytic glaucoma is caused by obstruction of trabecular meshwork with macrophages scavenged lens protein released through distended and weakened lens capsule.

Intraoperative Considerations

Absence of red reflex and poor visibility of the lens capsule make the surgery most challenging. Capsular staining is the most important tool in

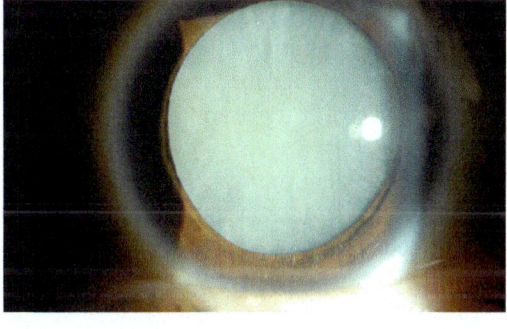

Fig. 1.1 Slit lamp photograph of intumescent cataract

W.S. Kim, K.H. Kim, *Challenges in Cataract Surgery*, DOI 10.1007/978-3-662-46092-4_1

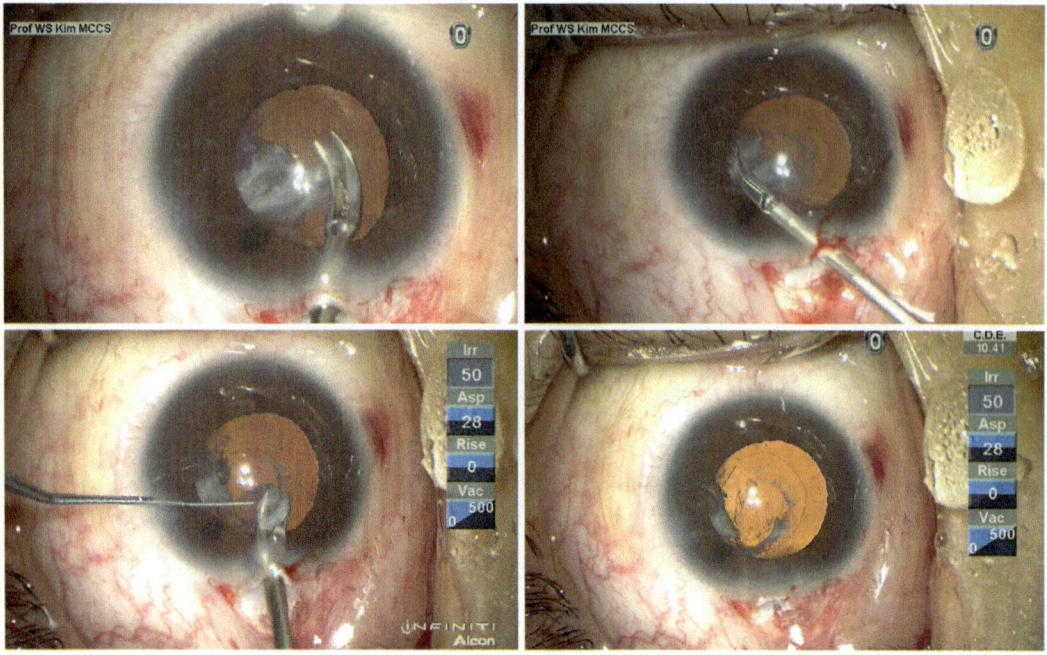

Fig. 1.2 Capsular plaque removal. Capsular scissors of various kinds can be utilized to cut across the plaques

managing the anterior capsule in the absence of red reflex.

Capsular Staining

For capsular staining, air is injected into the anterior chamber through the side port incision. The dye is injected under the air bubble using 27G blunt needle through side port incision. Trypan blue (Vision Blue®, DORC, Zuidland, Holland) is most frequently used in my practice because of its endothelial safety and effectiveness. Trypan blue is used to stain the anterior capsule during surgery and left to be in contract with the lens capsule for 1 min, then washed with BSS. Then is replaced with viscoelastics (Fig. 1.3 and 1.4).

Capsule staining can be performed by injecting dye on the surface of the capsule while the anterior chamber is filled with viscoelastics (preferably Healon5®, Pharmacia, Sweden). To perform this technique, anterior chamber should be maintained during injection of the dye into anterior chamber (Fig. 1.5).

Presence of zonular defect should be known before injection of trypan blue, because if it is leaked into the vitreous, it will diminish the red reflex even after removal of the lens material. I prefer to use Trypan blue in air-filled anterior chamber in order to prevent dilution of dye and provide homogenisty of the stain while minimize its contact with corneal endothelium.

Fluorescein sodium 2 % as well as methylene blue and gentian violet are also used. To use Fluoscein sodium cobalt blue illumination is necessary. Latter two are toxic to corneal endothelium and contact to endothelium should be monitored.

Tensions on the capsule make the capsulorhexis difficult and unpredictable.

Capsulorhexis more controllable with capsule staining and usage of viscoadaptive or dispersive viscoelastics by relieving the tensions on the capsule sufficiently. I prefer to use viscoadaptive viscoelastics because it can be readily removed at the completion of the surgery. Capsular staining coat the capsule and decrease the elasticity and usage of the viscoelastics push the anteriorly

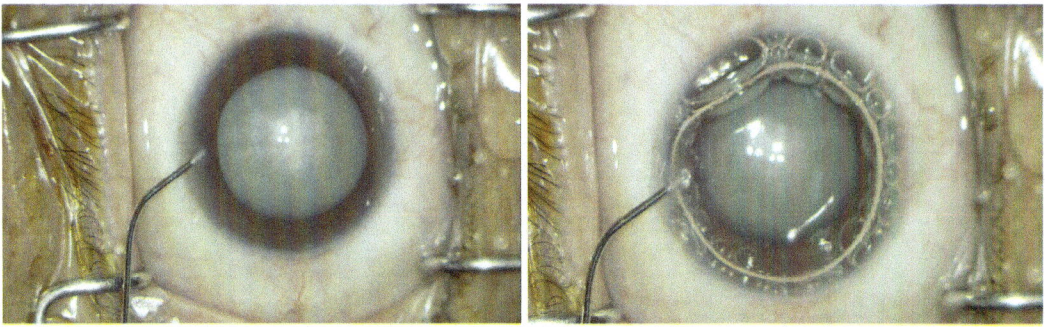

Fig. 1.3 (*Left*) Capsular staining procedures. Air syringe is inserted in anterior chamber through side port incision. (*Right*) Air is injected into anterior chamber through paracentesis. The big air bubble was made

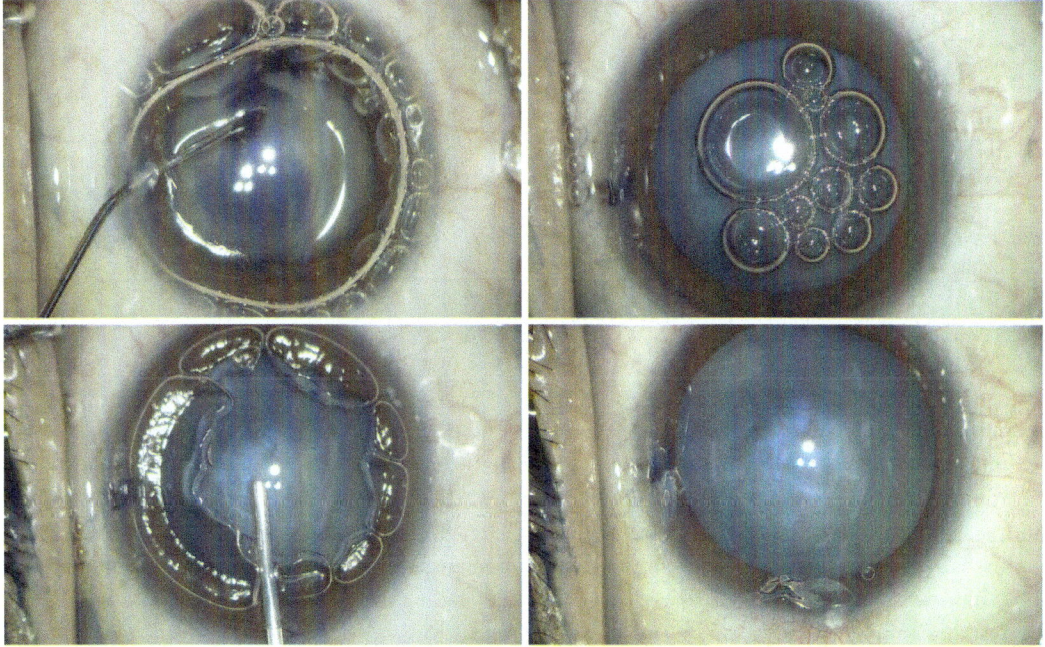

Fig. 1.4 (*Top Left*) Methlyene Blue is injected under the air bubble using 27G blunt needle through paracentesis. (*Top Right*) BSS is injected into anterior chamber to wash out dye. (*Bottom Left and Right*) Viscoelastics is injected into anterior chamber to to stabilize chamber and facilitated capsulorhexis

distended capsule posteriorly and decrease the tension on the capsule.

Capsulorhexsis

Capsulorhexis is performed but aim to create a smaller circle to prevent radial tear. Sometimes repeated injections of viscoelatics are necessary, however, too much injections of the viscoelas- tics that push the capsule behind the zonular plane will increase the tension on the capsule and make the capsulorhexis even more chal- lenging. Making an intact capsulorhexis is important in this case, because of the weak cap- sule, weak zonules and liquefied lens protein easily make the lens capsule lose its' integrity (radial tear and posterior capsule rupture) and even the implantation of the lens could be diffi- cult. Conversion to can-opener anterior capsu-

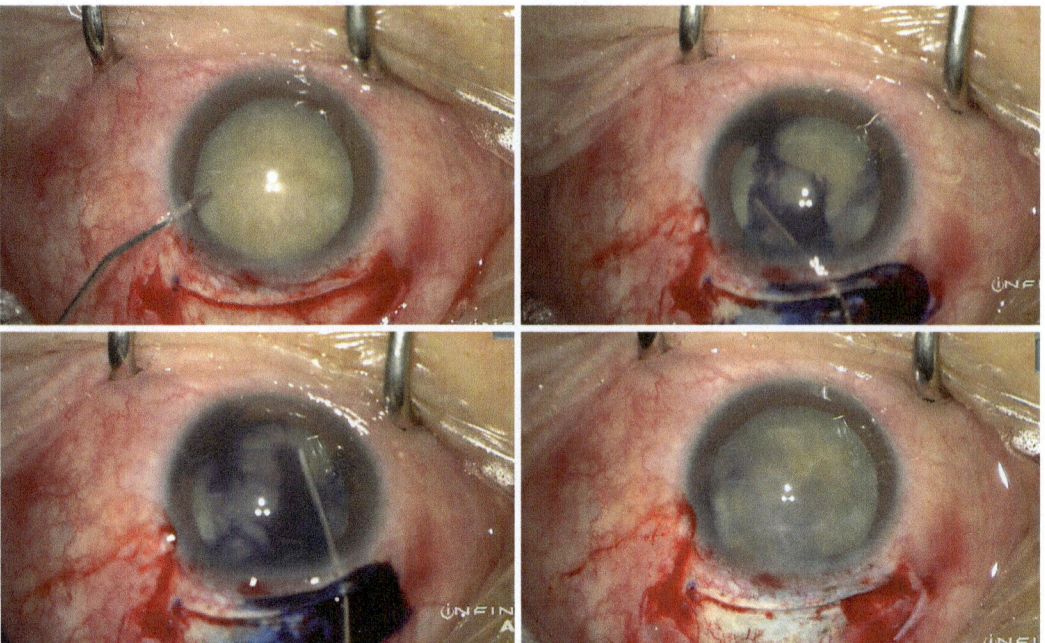

Fig. 1.5 Capsule staining can be performed by injecting dye on the surface of the capsule while the anterior chamber is filled with viscoelastics. (*Top Left*) Viscoelastics is injected into anterior chamber. (*Top Right* and *Bottom* *Left*) Methlyene Blue is injected under the viscoelastics. (*Bottom Right*) BSS is injected into anterior chamber to wash out dye and viscoelastics is reinjected

lotomy is an option when capsulorhexis cannot be finished as planned.

Another approach to improve visualization of the anterior capsule in the absence of the red reflex is "oblique illumination" using fibrotic light pipe can be used.

Another important characteristic of intumescent lens is thinned and stretched capsule that can be easily brought up to the phaco tip and break during phacoemulsification and also during I&A. During I&A, it is sometimes difficult to identify the presence of capsular tear and zonular dialysis in distended flaccid capsule. My preference of viscodissection is used by injecting cohesive viscoelastics between lens cortex and capsule (Fig. 1.6).

In the presence of capsular tear or zonular dialysis, removal of dispersive viscoelastics is difficult and damaging to the eye, however, dispersive viscoelastics are more convenient when separating the flaccid capsule from cortical material, they tend to stay with the capsule during I&A keeping the flaccid capsule away from the I&A tip, then risk of the capsule rupture can be decreased. Surgeon should consider these factors depending on the procedures he is taking (Fig. 1.7 and 1.8).

Intumescent cataract in young patients, consists only of liquefied materials, they are removed with I&A device. If there's any sign of zonular weakness, do not hesitate to use iris retractors to stabilize the capsule (retract the iris and CCC margin together) (Fig. 1.6).

If the nucleus density is high and capsule is weak such as in elderly patients, I prefer to perform iris plane phacoemulsification. Continuous phaco-emulsification can shallow the capsular bag and create a capsular tear, and also make corneal burn. There should be pauses between continuous phacoemulsification long enough to

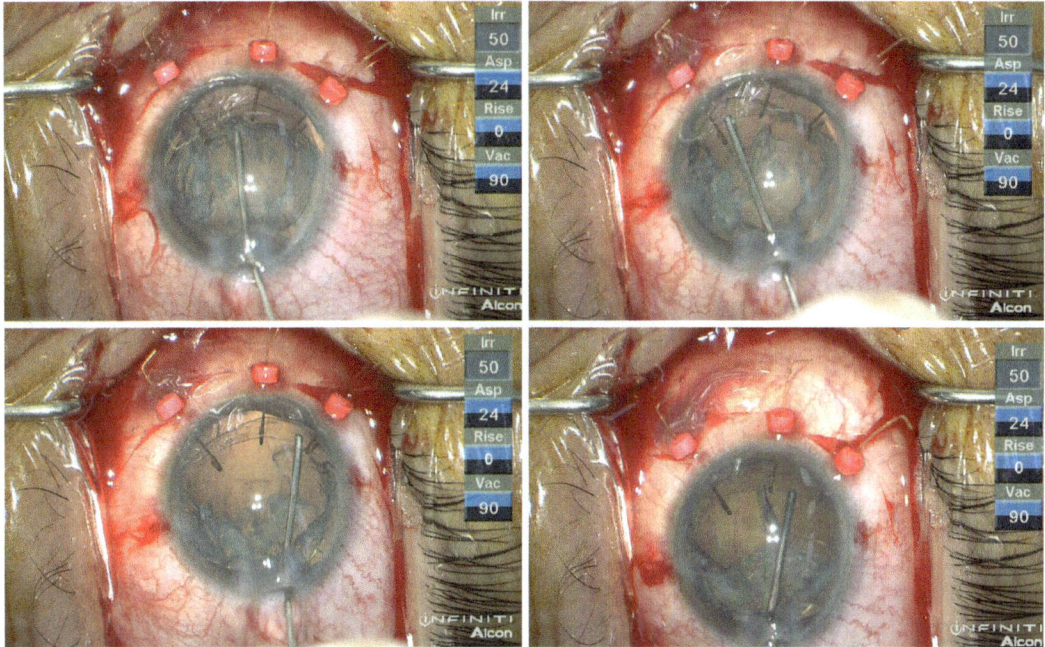

Fig. 1.6 Viscodissection, injecting cohesive viscoelastics between lens cortex and capsule was performed

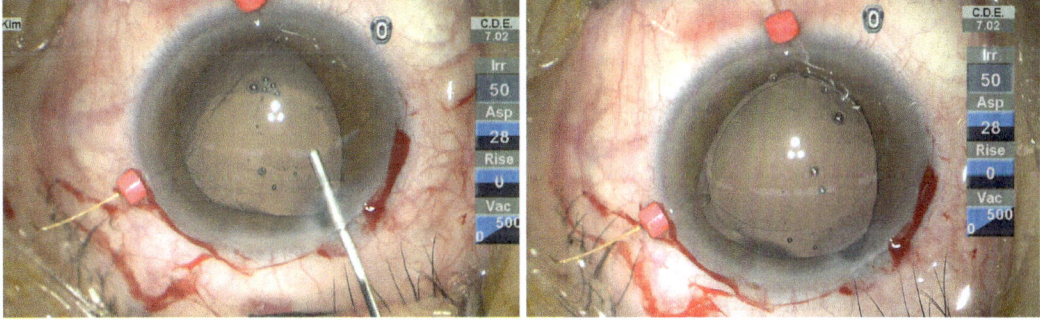

Fig. 1.7 (*Left*) Before Healon 5 injection, anterior chamber is collapsed. (*Right*) After Healon 5 injction, anterior chamber is filled with Healon 5

prevent bag shrinking and corneal burn. Because there is no protective cushion effect of epinucleus or cortex, during phaco emulsification, injection of viscoadaptive or dispersive viscoelastics behind the lens nucleus can help to hold the flaccid capsule and slow the movement of lens nucleus and prevent severe rubbing of lens nucleus against the posterior capsule.

Capsulorhexis is enlarged before implantation of IOL. Fill the capsular bag with viscoelastic. Too much distension of the bag should be avoided. I prefer to make a capsular scissors to make an initial cut. After grasping the flap using a capsular forceps, enlarge the initial capsulorhexis. IOL is implanted in the bag. My preference for this case is PMMA haptic foldable acrylic lens. In cases

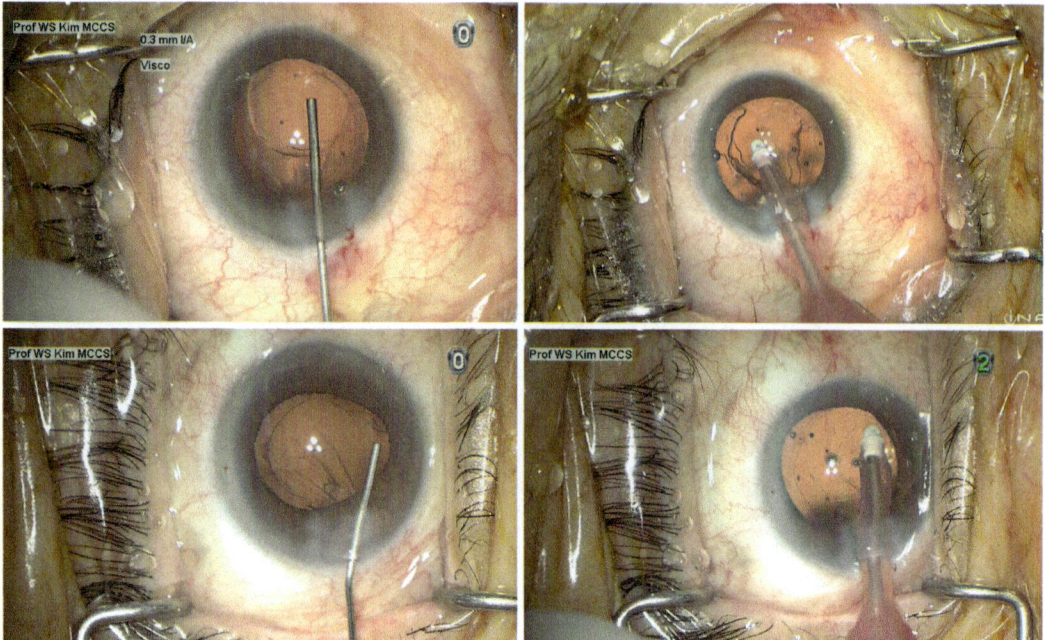

Fig. 1.8 (*Top Left*) Injection of visco-dispersive OVD into anterior chamber was done. (*Top Right*) Removal of visco-dispersive OVD using I&A is more time consuming as viscodipersive OVD tends to stay in the capsule.

(*Bottom Left*) Injection of visco-cohesive OVD into anterior chamber was done. (*Bottom Right*) Visco-cohesive OVD is easier to remove

with excessively distended capsular bag, IOLs are freely moving in the capsular bag.

In weak zonule cases, capsular contraction can occur relentlessly when CCC was not enlarged enough before completion of the surgery, careful follow up and YAG Laser anterior capsulotomy is required during follow up. In cases with severe zonular weakness or defect see Chaps. 10 and 11.

Postoperative Considerations

Postoperatively IOP rise can be frequent if visco-elastic was not removed completely (especially with dispersive viselastics), closer follow up IOP rise during immediate postop. is needed. In cases with loose zonules, IOL stability and capsule contracture should be evaluated at each postoperative visit.

Postop Medication

- Topical broad spectrum antibiotic: (levo-floxacin 0.5 % [Cravit®, Santen, Japan] or moxifloxacin 0.5 % [Vigamox®, Alcon, USA] qid)
- Topical steroids: (prednisolone acetate 1 % [Pred forte®, Allergan, USA] qid)
- Topical NSAIDs: (bromfenac [Bronuck®, Taejoon pharm., Korea] bid or flurbi-profen sodium 0.03 % [Flurbiprofen®, Basch&Lomb, USA] qid)
- May require treatment of increased intra-ocular pressure: dorzolamide/timolol [Cosopt®, Santen, Japan] bid, brimo-nidine tartrate 0.1 % [Alphagan-P®, Allergan, USA] bid, Carbonic anhydrase inhibitor, acetazolamide [Acetazol®, Hanlim pharm., Korea]

In mature cataract (Fig. 2.1), size of the lens is large, anterior chamber is shallow, possibility of weak zonules is present. There is little or no soft cortical material between hard nucleus and capsule, little or no red reflex, so is the safety margin. Especially in not experienced surgeon, possibility of conversion to ECCE should be considered beforehand. To accomplish successful phacoemulsification in dense cataract, there are several preparations and procedures that should be taken.

Preoperative Considerations

In dense cataract, careful history taking is important because, serious incidents affected the cataract eye might give other surgeons reasons to delay the operation. Retinal or optic nerve damage that might have occurred before could be the reason for the delay of the surgery, or findings such as phacodonesis that occur after a trauma gave a reason for the delay, therefore, there are possibilities of surgical challenges during the surgeries, and also possibilities of poor visual outcome after the surgeries. Careful history taking will give us the clue to the present cataract and future vision.

Intraoperative Considerations

If longer operation is anticipated, "pin point anesthesia" is performed before the surgery. I try to perform large capsulorhexis whenever possible for the better manipulation of dense nucleus when there is less room inside the capsular bag for in large dense cataract. Poor visibility of the capsule due to lack of red reflex can make capsulorhexis more challenging. Advance technologies in surgical microscope enabled us in better visualizing anterior capsule with no red reflex, sometimes, oblique external light source such as endoilluminator can be utilized [1, 2]. Capsular staining is a routine procedure in my practice for dense cataract, for better visualization and to add maneuverability to the fragile capsule by thickening the capsule and also by decreasing the elasticity of the capsule.

Dispersive or viscoadaptive viscoelastic is preferred to protect the cornea because they tend to adhere to the corneal endothelium and do not washed away to protect the endothelium, and because surgery is prolonged with multiple manipulations and more ultrasound energy is often employed to conquer hard nucleus.

Hydrodissection is difficult or often impossible due to the dense lens texture.

Cortical cleaving hydrodelineation is important to better maneuver the lens during lens removal. Multiple injections of small amount of BSS are given between CCC margin and the large dense nucleus to prevent "capsular block syndrome" [3, 4].

Small CCC increase the possibility of "capsular block syndrome" because the injected fluid is more easily flocculated behind the lens nucleus. By rocking the Nucleus sideways, fluid can be

W.S. Kim, K.H. Kim, *Challenges in Cataract Surgery*, DOI 10.1007/978-3-662-46092-4_2

dispersed around the large nucleus. Complete cortical cleaving hydrodissection is important to

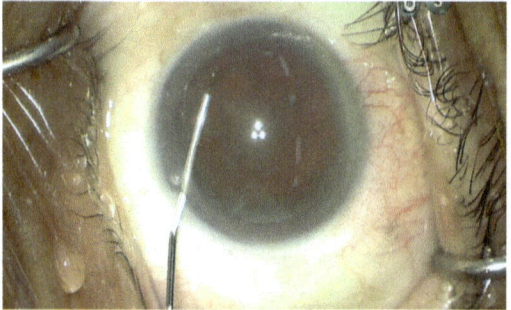

Fig. 2.1 Brunescent cataract with subtle retinal reflex is found

perform safe lens removal. If surgeon has difficulty completing the hydrodissection, one can do it later after the bulk of the nucleus has been removed.

"Divide and Conquer", "Stop and Chop" and various kinds of chopping techniques can be performed. As the size of the nucleus is big, nucleus better be divided into multiple small pieces. Be sure to insert phaco chopper under the CCC margin when lens cortex is little. When dividing the nucleus, fragment should be divided completely for quadrants to be removed.

The lens fibers especially located on the posterior side tend to be more tenacious and leathery. Sometimes, cutting the leathery part which is

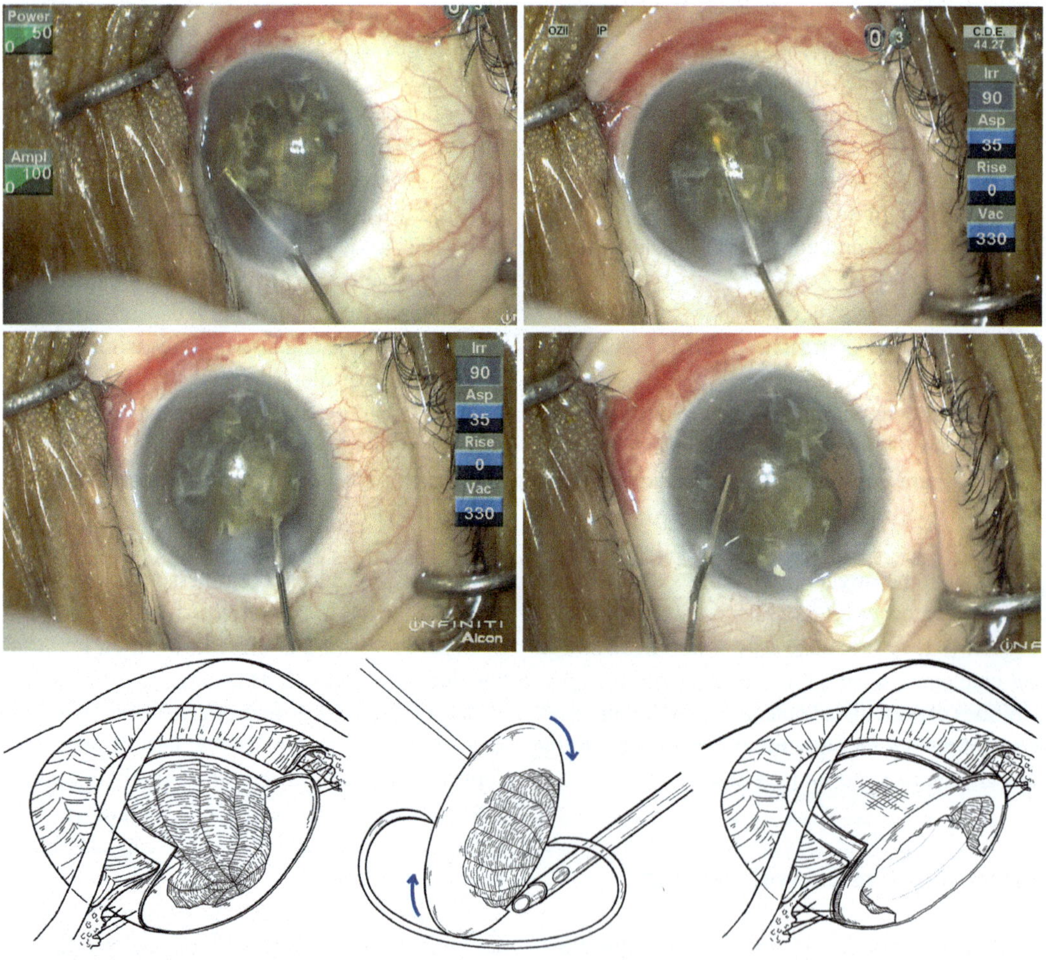

Fig. 2.2 (*Top Left*, *Top Right* and *Middle Left*) To remove the leathery posterior part of the lens, flipping the lens upside down is performed. Chopper is introduced through paracen-

tesis incision, then place it between the leathery stands. (*Middle Right*) Viscodissection is performed. (*Bottom*) Schematic illustrations of flipping the lens upside down

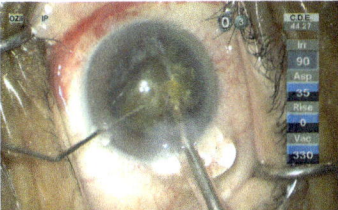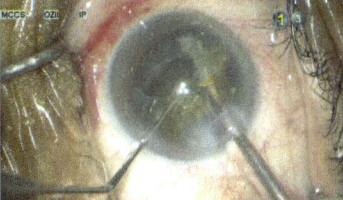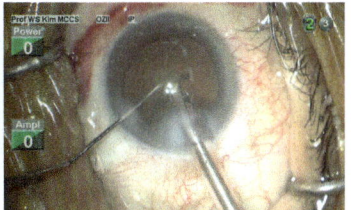

Fig. 2.3 Nucleus chopping is performed using chopper and phaco tip

located deepest posteriorly could be difficult and manual separation using chopper after elevation with viscoelastic is advised. To cut the leathery strands, if the volume of the lens is decreased enough, it could be easier to remove the leathery posterior part of the lens by flipping the lens upside down (Figs. 2.2 and 2.3). While holding the nucleus with the phaco tip, chopper is introduced through paracentesis incision, then place it between the leathery stands then pull it parallel toward the phaco tip. During phacoemulsification, injection of dispersive or viscoadaptive viscoelastics between posterior capsule and lens nucleus can keep the posterior capsule from touching the serrated edges of the dense nucleus.

When serrated edge of the hard nucleus rubs against the posterior capsule during phacoemulsification, then posterior capsule will rupture readily because there is no protective layer between posterior capsule and lens nucleus. Be sure to keep the serrated margin of the hard nucleus away from the posterior capsule. Increase the phaco power as the density of the lens nucleus increases.

As with the advancements in technologies has decreased the phaco energy consumption greatly, hence the phaco tip temperature and corneal incisional burns. However still, the incidence of the corneal burn [5] is highest in cases with rock hard nucleus, I advise to take pauses between continuous phacoemulsifications. When prolonged phaco time is expected, for prevention of corneal endothelium damage, use of dispersive viscoelastics

are desired, they are not flushed out of the anterior chamber in seconds during manipulation.

To make less fluctuation of anterior chamber with minimal leak during capsulorhexis, dispersive viscoelastics or "soft shell technique" [6] provides comfortable atmosphere to surgeon, however, volume effect and visualizationis better with cohesive viscoelastics. During phacoemulsification, dispersive viscoelastics can provide barrier between hard nucleus and the fragile capsule because they are not removed readily. During lens implantation, cohesive viscoelastic is used because they are easier to be removed.

Postoperative Considerations

Postoperative IOP (Intraocular Pressure) spike is not uncommon due to remained viscoelastics or cortical nuclear fragments, medical treatment is usually adequate, but anterior chamber irrigation can be needed occasionally.

Corneal edema is common, because too much ultrasound energy is delivered during phacoemulsification. Topical 5 % NaCl is uses four times a day to alleviate corneal edema. Corneal wound burn causes corneal distortion, astigmatism, and wound disruption. Sometimes require corneal suture or glue can be applied when appropriate wound construction cannot be achieved [7, 8].

Postop Medication

- Topical broad spectrum antibiotic: (levofloxacin 0.5 % [Cravit®, Santen, Japan] or moxifloxacin 0.5 % [Vigamox®, Alcon, USA] qid)
- Topical steroids: (prednisolone acetate 1 % [Pred forte®, Allergan, USA] qid)
- Topical NSAIDs: (bromfenac [Bronuck®, Taejoon pharm., Korea] bid or flurbiprofen sodium 0.03 % [Flurbiprofen®, Basch&Lomb, USA] qid) - May require treatment of increased intraocular pressure: (dorzolamide/timolol [Cosopt®, Santen, Japan] bid, brimonidine tartrate 0.1 % [Alphagan-P®, Allergan, USA] bid, Carbonic anhydrase inhibitor, acetazolamide [Acetazol®, Hanlim pharm., Korea]

References

1. Takkar B, Azad R, Azad S, Rathi A. Posterior segment nucleotomy for dislocated sclerotic cataractous lens using chandelier endoilluminator and sharp tipped chopper. Int J Ophthalmol. 2015;8:833–4.
2. Matalia J, Anaspure H, Shetty BK, Matalia H. Intraoperative usefulness and postoperative results of the endoilluminator for performing primary posterior capsulectomy and anterior vitrectomy during pediatric cataract surgery. Eye (Lond). 2014;28:1008–13.
3. Yip CC, Au Eong KG, Yong VS. Intraoperative capsular block syndrome masquerading as expulsive hemorrhage. Eur J Ophthalmol. 2002;12:333–5.
4. Updegraff SA, Peyman GA, McDonald MB. Pupillary block during cataract surgery. Am J Ophthalmol. 1994;117:328–32.
5. Syed ZA, Moayedi J, Mohamedi M. Cataract surgery outcomes at a UK independent sector treatment centre. Br J Ophthalmol. 2015;99:1460–5.
6. Arshinoff SA. Dispersive-cohesive viscoelastic soft shell technique. J Cataract Refract Surg. 1999;25:167–73.
7. Vote BJ, Elder MJ. Cyanoacrylate glue for corneal perforations: a description of a surgical technique and a review of the literature. Clin Experiment Ophthalmol. 2000;28:437–42.
8. Fynn-Thompson N, Goldstein MH. Management of corneal thinning, melting, and perforation. In: Yanoff M, Duker J. Ophthalmology. 4th ed. Saunders, 2014; Chap. 2, pp 325–7.

Characteristics of uveitis cataract are presence of underlying systemic disease, poor tolerance to IOL, technical difficulty in cataract surgery due to maturity in cataract caused by deferred surgery, iris deformity, synechiae, and high rate of perioperative complications (such as glaucoma, uveitis and synechiae) (Fig. 3.1).

Preoperative Considerations

Control of underlying systemic disease should be considered before surgery. Multidisciplinary approach is needed to control the systemic inflammation. Often the surgery is delayed due to many reasons (hesitation by the surgeon and the patient, referral to another clinic, control of inflammation…), it is hard to determine the status of the posterior pole. Therefore, other measures such as potential acuity meter or laser interferometry are often used for the evaluation of potential visual outcome after the surgery.

For evaluation of postoperative visual outcome, pre-existing conditions that might occur due to uveitis should be evaluated (such as, cystoid macular edema, epiretinal membrane, optic neuropathy). Consultation is needed with retina specialist for the treatment of certain patients with retinal complications. Retinal optical coherence tomography (OCT) has been a routine preoperative evaluation of retina before cataract surgery in our practice.

The causes of uveitis should be evaluated whenever possible, because, the cause of the disease can determine the prognosis. Laboratory evaluation and consultation with Rheumatologists are routinely done.

Use of intraocular lens is a controversy in some conditions such as juvenile rheumatoid arthritis, Vogt-Koyanagi-Harada syndrome, sympathetic ophthalmia, or recurrent granulomatous uveitis of any cause with extensive synechiae formation.

IOL selection is another challenge for the surgeon. The design, overall diameter, and configurations of the IOL are huge concerns. I prefer to choose intraocular lens that does not touch the uveal tissue once placed in the capsular bag. I also prefer intraocular lens that does not deformed by contracting capsular bag that occurs after uveitis cataract surgery. Prolene was accused of activation of complement when in contact with metabolically active tissue. IOL should be tried to be placed in the bag where touching of the uveal tissue is minimum. Posterior chamber lenses designed for and placed in the capsular bag could reduce the mechanical irritation.

Proper control of intraocular pressure is needed, however, cholinergic drugs should not be used because they tend to increase the synechiae formation, by altering aqueous barrier. I try not to use prostaglandin analogue not to activate complement pathway.

In uveitis cataract patient, more than 3 months of inflammation free period is required to assure successful surgery. In long-standing uveitis, flare cannot be eliminated completely, control of

© Springer-Verlag Berlin Heidelberg 2016
W.S. Kim, K.H. Kim, *Challenges in Cataract Surgery*, DOI 10.1007/978-3-662-46092-4_3

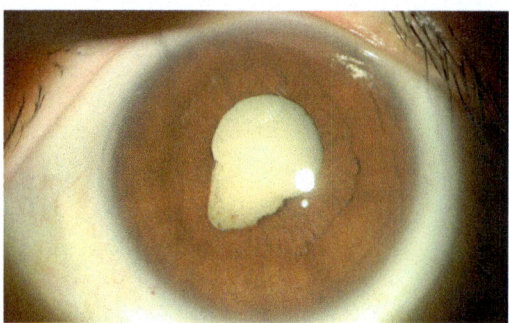

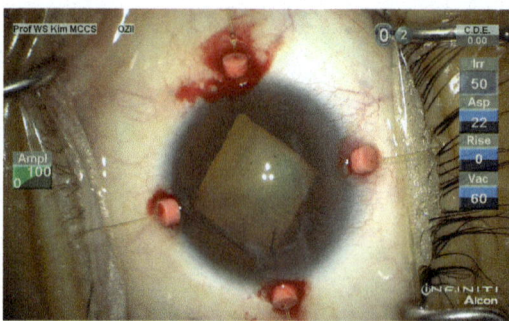

Fig. 3.1 Slit lamp photogragh of uveitis cataract. Posterior synechiae is visible on inferior quadrant

Fig. 3.2 Iris retractors are inserted to make sufficient pupillary dilation

active anterior chamber cells or vitreous cells is required. The mainstay of preoperative anti-inflammatory therapy is topical corticosteroids. Strong topical corticosteroids, such as prednisolone 1 % is given eight times a day starting 1 weeks before surgery. One mg/kg/day or oral prednisone (usually 60–80 mg) is given for 1 week before surgery. Topical and systemic use of nonsteroidal anti-inflammatory drugs has been used by some surgeon in cases of cystoid macular edema or without proven efficacy.

There are cases when cataract surgery should be performed in an eye with active uveitis; in cases have disabling visual impairment with inflammations not completely controlled with any medication, or cases when urgent vitreoretinal surgery is required which cannot be performed without cataract surgery. Intraorbital injection of corticosteroids and oral prednisolone is used. Imunosuppressive agent use is considered, consultation to rheumatologist is needed [1–3].

Intraoperative Considerations

Topical anesthesia is enough most of the cases, however, pinpoint anesthesia, peribulbar or retrobulbar anesthesia is preferred when iris manipulation is expected.

Good pupillary dilation is needed to minimize iris touching during surgery. Use of mechanical dilation using iris retractor is required when proper dilation is not achieved pharmacologically. Before using stretching devices, fibrous ring covering the pupillary margin should be

transected using scissors or stripped off using capsulorhexhis forceps to allow traction of the pupillary margin radially. During scissoring, caution should be used not to cut the iris vessels. During stretching of the iris minimal trauma should be exerted to the iris, extreme traction can cause hemorrhage, permanent pupil dilation, and severe postoperative inflammation.

Small clear corneal incision, and phacoemulsification are preferred by many surgeons. It reduces inflammation, iris trauma during lens manipulation. Short scleral tunnel incision is preferred when implantation of a rigid PMMA lens is planned. Posterior synechiae should be lysed gently using round spatula placed between lens capsule and iris. Stretching the pupil using two hooked instruments (IOL manipulator or Sinskey hook) 180° apart can help to break the circumferential fibrous band. Epinephrine containing balanced salt solution can dilate the pupil at this stage. If the dilation is not sufficient to performed safe surgery or iris is too floppy, it is best to use iris retractor (Fig. 3.2).

In uveitis cataract, I prefer not to perform sphinterotomies or radial iridotomy which can cause severe postoperative inflammation. Likewise, I prefer not to perform peripheral iridectomy during surgery unless the risk of development of iris bombe is high. However, if pupils are not reacting when active inflammation is anticipated, surgical iridectomy is performed because the patency rate is higher in surgical iridectomy than using the YAG laser.

Size of CCC margin is important because inflamed eye causes more aggressive capsule contraction, CCC margin should be large enough to prevent capsule contraction and following in –the-bag IOL dislocation. If CCC cannot be made large enough, two radial incisions can be made on CCC margin, 180° apart (CCC can be enlarged using YAG laser capsulotomy, however, when iris cannot be enlarged pharmaceutically, CCC should be enlarged before completion of the surgery).

Selection of IOL could also be critical. If IOL's haptic cannot resist the contracting capsular bag, same thing happens. During removal of the nucleus and cortical material iris damage should be minimized to prevent postoperative inflammation. All the lens materials should be removed meticulously.

I prefer to make large capsulorhexis, which will not cause capsule contraction at a later date. Capsulorhexis in uveitis eye is less challenging because the capsule is less elastic and more controllable than that of the normal cataract patient. I also prefer to perform posterior capsulorhexis with optic capturing, however, in the bag IOL placement was enough in most of the cases.

Phaco chop is my preferred technique for removal of hard nucleus. Intensive cortical clean up is critical to eliminated major source of postoperative inflammatory reaction. All the capsular bag should be inspected thoroughly by retracting the pupillary margin, not to leave any cortical material behind. Suturing of the incision is adviced by some surgeons. Pupil may be dilated or constricted at the completion of the surgery (constricted for large capsulorhexis, dilated for small capsulorhexis). Topical and subconjunctival corticosteroids are administered at the completion of the surgery. Intravitreal corticosteroid use has been reported to be useful in selected cases such as juvenile idiopathic arthritis and intolerance to systemic corticosteroid [4].

Combined pars plana vitrectomy and lensectomy are preferred by vitreoretinal surgeons and must be considered when posterior segment disease must be surgically treated.

In cases with Juvenile Rheumatoid Arthritis cases, even after IOL optic capturing through PCCC (posterior capsulorhexis), iridocapsular and peripheral anterior synechiae was unavoidable. Membranes grow over the IOL on anterior and posterior surface. There are advocates for the

removal of lens through a limbal approach and advocates of a pars plana approach for JRA to prevent lens capsules scaffolding and cyclitic membrane formation. Lens implantation is not recommended for these cases [5].

This surgery is most frequently considered in patients with juvenile rheumatoid arthritis and pars planitis. IOLs are poorly indicated in this case. Posterior capsule is removed completely to prevent scaffolding for cyclitic membrane. If IOL is implanted, it is implanted in the sulcus anterior to the residual anterior capsule.

Combined phacoemulsification and pars plana vitrectomy technique has many advantages. IOL can be placed in the bag for the purpose of minimal uveal tissue contact and faster visual rehabilitation.

Selection of IOL is an important issue in the surgery of uveitis cataract. PMMA lens has advantages over prolene, because prolen is known to activate complement cascade and be related to higher incidence of endophthalmitis. Silicon lenses, PMMA lenses and Acrylic lenses are well tolerated. Acrylic foldable IOL is my preferred IOL for this occasion because it can be folded to be inserted through small corneal incision and does not cause serious inflammatory reaction, Surface modified IOLs have theoretical advantages in uveitis cataract. Foldable IOL with PMMA haptic to prevent capsule contraction especially when zonules are weak or CCC is not large enough. I also prefer to use IOLs with angulation to minimize the contact between the IOL and the iris. Anterior chamber IOL is contraindicated due to expected serious inflammation.

I always place the IOL in the bag whenever more than moderate amount of active inflammation is anticipated, although sulcus fixated IOL are reported to well tolerated in many occasions. Sulcus placement and anterior chamber placement can increase the rubbing of IOL against uveal tissue resulting in chronic inflammation and iris atrophy. I prefer to capture the IOL optic through PCCC in order to compartmentalize the vitreous cavity from anterior chamber which is inflamed immediate postoperative period. Optic capturing also prevent development of PCO which is frequent after uveitis cataract surgery (Figs. 3.3, 3.4, and 3.5).

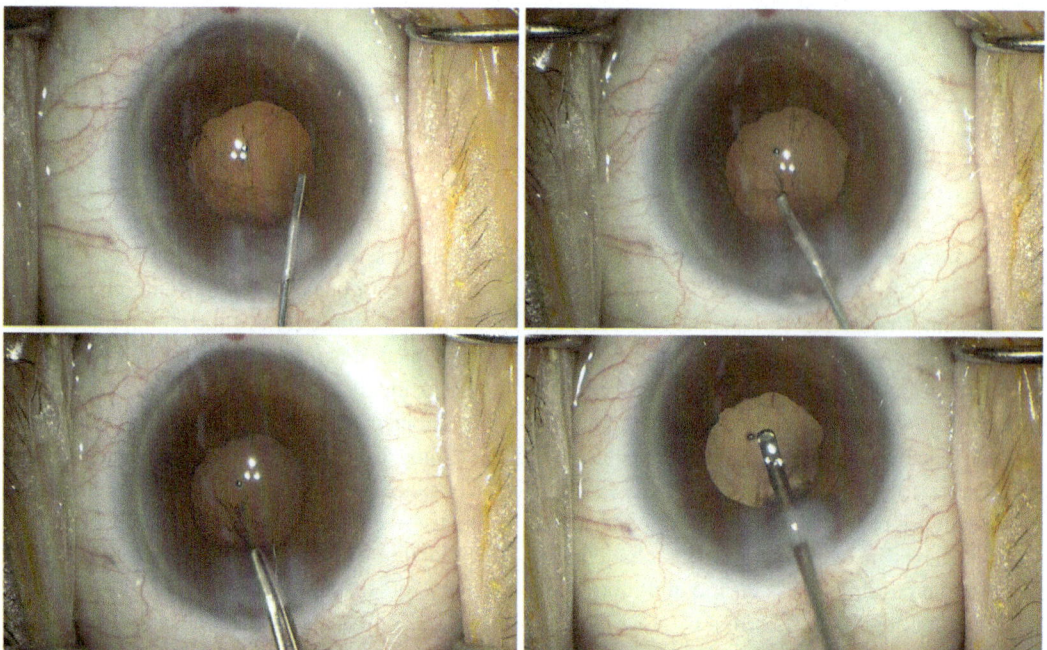

Fig. 3.3 (*Top Left*) OVD is injected into anterior chamber. (*Top Right*) Posterior lens capsule puncture is done with puncture needle (*Bottom Left*) PCCC is done with capsular forcep. (*Bottom Right*) Dry anterior vitrectomy is performed with vitrectomy cutter to removed anterior vitreous to prevent vitreous prolapsed to anterior chamber

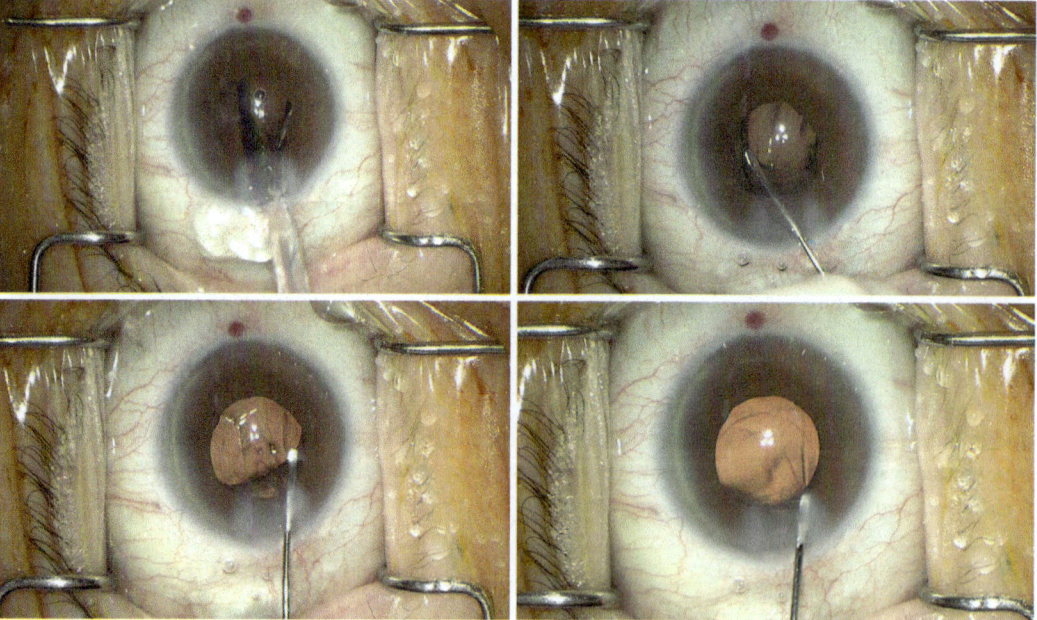

Fig. 3.4 (*Top Left*) 3-piece IOL is inserted in the bag. (*Top Right*) IOL is manipulated by rotator. (*Bottom Left and Right*) IOL optic capture is performed

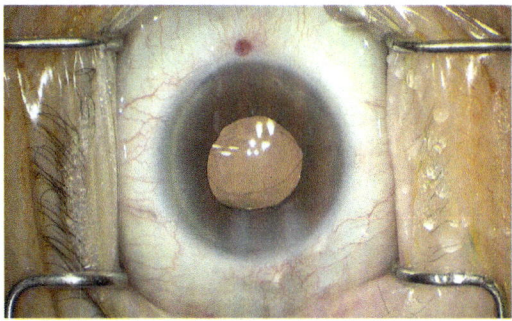

Fig. 3.5 IOL is capture to posterior capsule. Haptics are in the bag, Optic is under the capsule

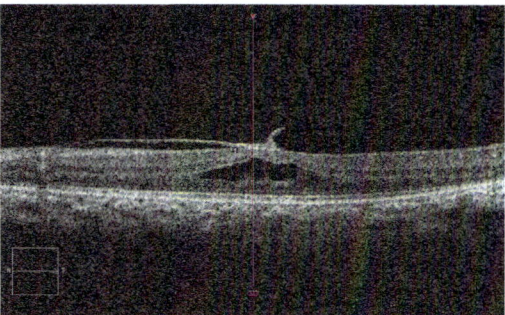

Fig. 3.6 Macular pucker in JRA patient. Foveal traction with thick fibrous membrane is found

If intraoperative surgical complication does not allow in the bag IOL placement, and the eye has been quiet for more than a year without medication, IOL placement in the sulcus or scleral fixation can be considered. When in-the–bag IOL placement of both eyes are not feasible in actively inflamed eye, patients having only one functioning eye, I'd rather leave the eye aphakic.

If membrane formation and active inflammation cannot be controlled medically after implantation of IOL in the sulcus, it should be removed.

After cataract surgery, occurence of vitreous opacification is frequent. Vitrectomy for shrunk opacified vitreous is not a challenge, and be performed through pars plana using a closed system. Dexamathasone subconjunctival injection is given at the completion of the surgery.

Postoperative Considerations

Strict control of inflammation is the key to successful surgery. Topical corticosteroids should be used every hour immediately after the operation then tapers down until 1–2 months. Oral prednisone 1 mg/kg/day for 7days then tapering it down slowly for a month. Topical nonsteroidal anti-inflammatory drops are used as a routine medication.

Incidence of posterior synechiae is high, when the capsulorhexis is large keep the pupil small, when the size of the capsulorhexis is small dilating the pupil was advocated to minimize the contact between posterior surface of the iris and capsulorhexis margin where the intial synechia begins. I prefer to use short acting mydriatics (PhyenylephrineHCl 5 mg/ml, Tropicamide

5 mg/ml) twice a day for 3–4 weeks to prevent synechiae formation.

If IOP is increased, beta blockers, dorzolamide, or systemic acetazolamide are used. Uncontrolled glaucoma will require filteration surgery. If inflammatory glaucoma and iris bombe was not avoidable YAG laser iridectomy or surgical iridectomy is performed.

Pupillary membrane can be removed surgically. Hypotony and Cyclitic membrane can occur in severe cases of uveitis, can be removed by pars plana vitrectomy and membranectomy. Macular pucker can occur (Fig. 3.6). Cystoid macular edema is the most serious postoperative complication in cases with long-standing uveitis [6–8]. When it develops postoperatively and does not respond to medical treatment refer to the retina specialist is needed for evaluation and surgical treatment.

Patients with chronic juvenile arthritis have exacerbation of the uveitis process after cataract surgery. Anterior vitrectomy is recommended by some surgeons [9, 10]. When surgery is performed in visually developing eye (younger than 8 years old/ greater amblyopia rick with youger age), amblyopia treatment should be done with careful monitoring of the postoperative inflammation, intraocular pressure, and changes in vision. They should be informed about greater risk of various complications and repeated surgery (eg. vitrectomy, membranectomy, glaucoma filtering).

For pediatric patients, since they are not cooperative enough to perform OCT or Visual Field, IOP measurement and portable fundus photography is needed to follow the changes in optic disc. There are useful labratory testing to identify the underlying conditions in Table 3.1.

Table 3.1 Laboratory test for uveitis

Laboratory tests	Associated disease
Blood chemistry panel	
Rheumatoid panel	Connective tissue diseases (RA, SLE, etc.)
Human leukocyte antigen (HLA) haplotypes	Spondyloarthropathies, behçet syndrome
Angiotensin-converting enzyme (ACE)	Sarcoidosis
Lysozyme	Sarcoidosis or tuberculosis
Antineutrophil cytoplasmic antibody lupus anticoagulant panel, total complement panel, protein electrophoresis	Connective tissue diseases
Treponemal and nontreponemal tests	Syphilis
Viral antibody testing	HSV, HZV, hepatitis, cytomegalovirus, or HIV
Chest radiograph	Tuberculosis or sarcoidosis
Tuberculin skin test	Tuberculosis
Behcetin skin test with hypodermic needle may also be considered.	
Lumbar, thoracic, and sacroiliac spine radiographs	Ankylosing spondylitis
Magnetic resonance imaging of the brain	Multiple sclerosis

Postop Medication

- Topical broad spectrum antibiotic : (levofloxacin 0.5 % [Cravit®, Santen, Japan] or moxifloxacin 0.5 % [Vigamox®, Alcon, USA] qid)
- Topical steroids : Strict control of inflammation is important (predniso-lone acetate 1 % [Pred forte®, Allergan, USA] up to 1 h)
- Oral prednisone 1 mg/kg/day for 7days then tapering it down for a month
- Topical NSAIDs : (bromfenac [Bronuck®, Taejoon pharm., Korea] bid or flurbipro-fen sodium 0.03 % [Flurbiprofen®, Basch & Lomb, USA] qid)

- Topical cycloplegics : (cyclopentolate 1 % [Ocucyclo®, Samil pharm, Korea], scopolamine 0.25 %, or atropine 1 % bid to qid depending on severity)
- May require treatment of increased intra-ocular pressure: dorzolamide/timolol [Cosopt®, Santen, Japan] bid, brimoni-dine tartrate 0.1 % [Alphagan-P®, Allergan, USA] bid, Carbonic anhydrase inhibitor, acetazolamide [Acetazol®, Hanlim pharm., Korea]

References

1. Wells JM, Smith JR. Uveitis in juvenile idiopathic arthritis: recent therapeutic advances. Ophthalmic Res. 2015;54:124–7.
2. Sadiq MA, Agarwal A, Hassan M, et al. Therapies in development for non-infectious uveitis. Curr Mol Med. 2015;15:565–77.
3. Cordero-Coma M, Salazar-Méndez R, Yilmaz T. Treatment of severe non-infectious uveitis in high-risk conditions (Part 2): systemic infections; manage-ment and safety issues. Expert Opin Drug Saf. 2015;14:1353–71.
4. Okhravi N, Morris A, Dowler GF, et al. Intraoperative use of intravitreal triamcinolone in uveitic eyes hav-ing cataract surgery: pilot study. J Cataract Refract Surg. 2007;33:1278–83.
5. Li J, Heinz C, Zurek-Imhoff B, Heiligenhaus A. Intraoperative intraocular triamcinolone injection prophylaxis for post-cataract surgery fibrin formation in uveitis associated with juvenile idiopathic arthritis. J Cataract Refract Surg. 2006;32:1535–9.
6. Ram J, Gupta A, Kumar S, et al. Phacoemulsification with intraocular lens implantation in patients with uveitis. J Cataract Refract Surg. 2010;36:1283–8.
7. Rahman I, Jones NP. Long-term results of cataract extraction with intraocular lens implantation in patients with uveitis. Eye. 2005;19:191–7.
8. Roesel M, Heinz C, Koch JM. Heiligen haus A. Cataract surgery in uveitis. Ophthalmology. 2008;115:1431.
9. Kotaniemi K, Penttila H. Intraocular lens implanta-tion in patients with juvenile idiopathic arthritis-associated uveitis. Ophthalmic Res. 2006;38:318–23.
10. Terrada C. Cataract surgery with primary intraocular lens implantation in children with uveitis: long-term outcomes. J Cataract Refract Surg. 2011;37:1977–83.

With the introduction of NSAID, incidence of constricting pupil has been decreased greatly, however, there are a lot of conditions that pupils would not dilate pharmacologically.

Pharmaceuticals

In our practice 0.5 % tropicamide and 0.5 % phenylephrine (Mydrin-P, Santen, Japan) is being used. Addition of higher concentration mydriatics are known to be effective in dilating the pupils. The use of preoperative anti-inflammatory agents (NSAIDs), such as flurbiprofensodium (Ocufen, Allergan, USA) or bronfenac sodium (Bronuck, Taejoon, Korea) decreased occasions of intraoperative pupillary constrictions greatly. Intracameral injection of 1:10,000 preservative free epinephrine or mixture of 1:100,000 epinephrine is being used at surgeons preference.

Ophthalmic Viscosurgical Devices (OVD)

I prefer to use viscoadaptic viscoelastics since they can push the iris plane and stay there for a while. Complete removal of viscoadaptive OVD is required because these eyes alreadily have higher risk for developing glaucoma.

Phaco Parameters

In small pupil phacoemulsification, high flow can increase the followability can increase the phaco efficiency, however, continuous phaco aspiration can easily collapse the anterior chamber. Interrupted phaco better be required and capsular bag distension must be continuously monitored.

Small Pupil Phacoemulsification

Even with not fully dilated pupil, phacoemulsification can be performed. With moderately dilated (3–5 mm in diameter) pupil, capsulorhexis can be made larger than the pupil size. Complete hydrodissection is needed to fully utilize the followability. I prefer to use Vertical Chopping technique (Fig. 4.1), however, any technique that we perform in center of the nucleus can be used.

In small pupil phacoemulsification, long continuous phacoemulsification should not be performed with the phaco tip placed in the bag. Because the irrigation flow is blocked by the small pupil and

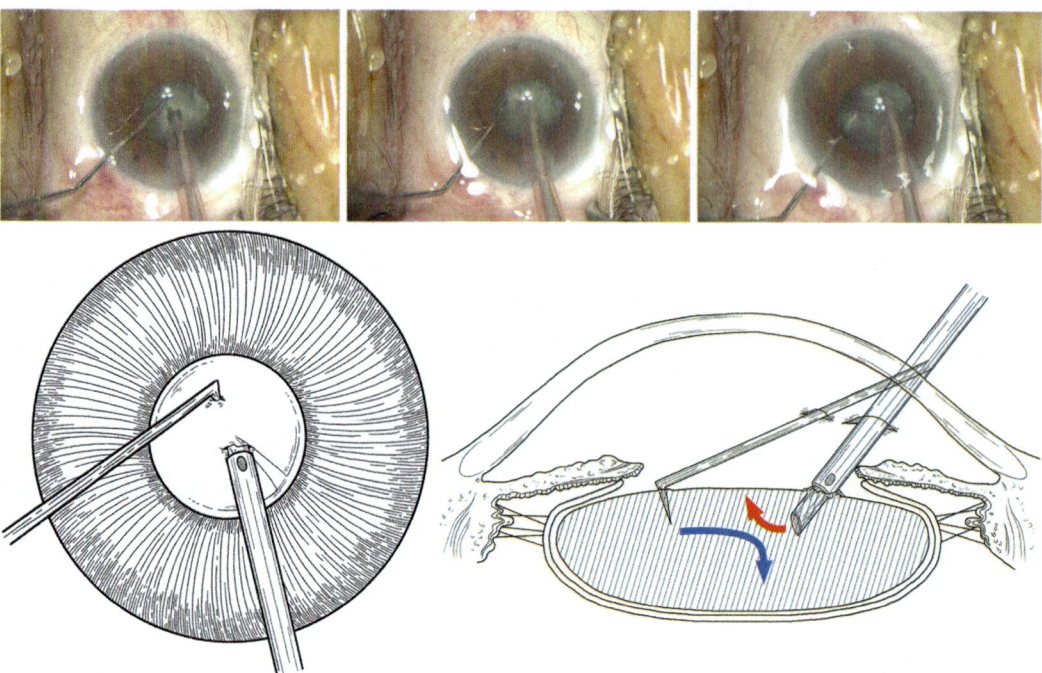

Fig. 4.1 (*Top Line*) Vetical chopping technique is performed to separate nucleus in small pupil phacoemulsification. (*Bottom line*) Schematic illustration for vertical chopping technique

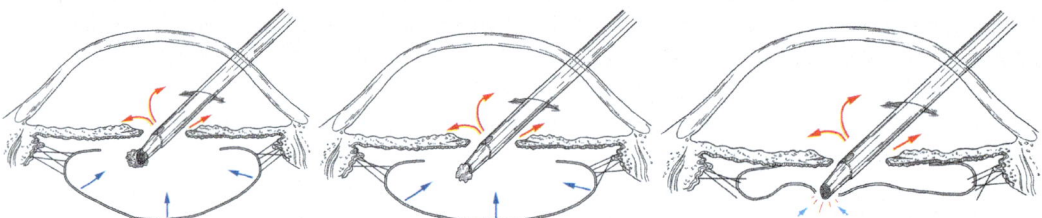

Fig. 4.2 If the irrigation flow is blocked by the small pupil and does not effectively fill the bag readily, aspiration and phacoemulsification can easily collapse the lens capsular bag then break the capsule

does not effectively fill the bag readily, aspiration and phacoemulsification can easily collapse the lens capsular bag then break the capsule (Fig. 4.2).

If corneal decompensation is not a matter, anterior chamber phaco-emulsification could be an option. Certain level of nuclear sclerosis and pupil dilation can be a limitation to perform phacoemulsification, therefore, we have to look for other measures to dilate the pupil to safely complete cataract surgery.

Pupil Dilation During Surgery (Fig. 4.4)

Stepwise Pupil Dilation

Stage 1. If I find fibrous membrane along and behind the pupillary margin, usually the miosis is due to restrictive constriction due to the fibrous membrane behind the pupil. Membrane should be removed to dilate the pupil using capsular forceps (Fig. 4.3). Pupil would dilate with injection of OVD injection into anterior chamber (Fig. 4.4).

Stage 2. If the pupil does not dilate after removal of the membrane, mechanical stretching with hooks such as Sinsky hook and Lens Manipulator with each hands could dilate the pupil (Excessive stretching that damage the pupillary sphincter should be avoided. If any sign of iris tear is found, stretching must be stopped) (Fig. 4.5).

Stage 3. If the pupil still does not dilate or if the dilated pupil is too floppy to perform phacoemulsificiation, I use iris retractors made of Prolene (Fig. 4.6).

There are various kinds of iris retractors. Iris retractors are safer in a way that they can control the amount of retraction. I prefer to use Prolene iris retractors than Metal ones. Former one is more controllable and less damaging to the ocular tissue during surgery. Latter ones tend to dislodge during surgery, risk of capsule tear is higher, however, less costly because they are usually reusable.

In placing stab incisions, I prefer to make limbal incisions rather than clear corneal one and make corneal passes parallel to the iris, to prevent iris tenting toward the cornea. Excessive tenting can easily damage the iris and should be avoided. I try to make small sized anterior chamber entry just enough to make entry and exit of the iris hooks possible to minimize aqueous leak from anterior chamber during surgery. I also prefer to place iris retractor under the corneal incision, because retracted iris on the quadrant of incision minimize the iris damage during surgery.

Extreme caution must be used when mechanically stretching the iris not to damage the sphincter pupillae muscle. Especially in cases with iris stromal atrophy (e.g., Leprosy), iris tear can happen seriously during stretching of the iris, during

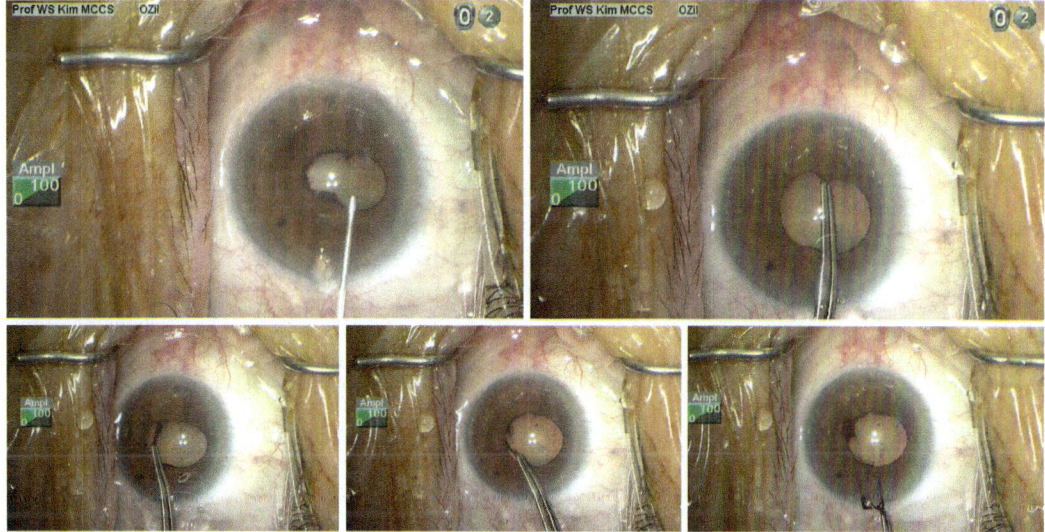

Fig. 4.3 (*Top Left*) Poor pupillary dilation with posterior synechiae are found in uveitis cataract patient. (*Top Right*) Retro-pupillary membrane is grasped with capsular for-ceps. (*Bottom Line*) Grasped pupillary membrane is peeled counter clockwise

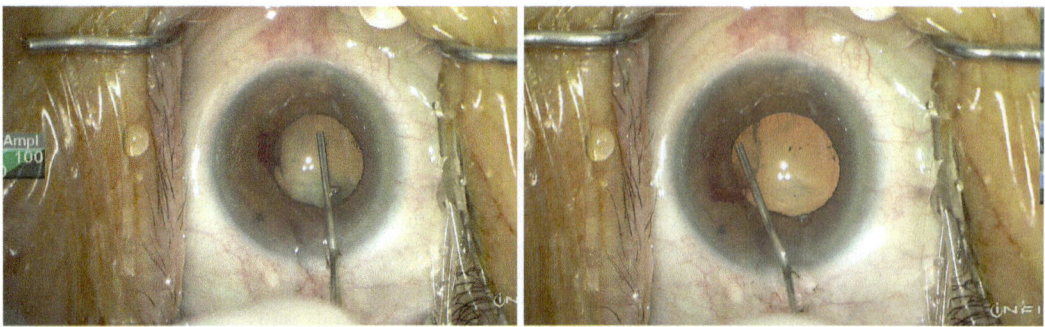

Fig. 4.4   Pupil would dilate with injection of OVD injection into anterior chamber

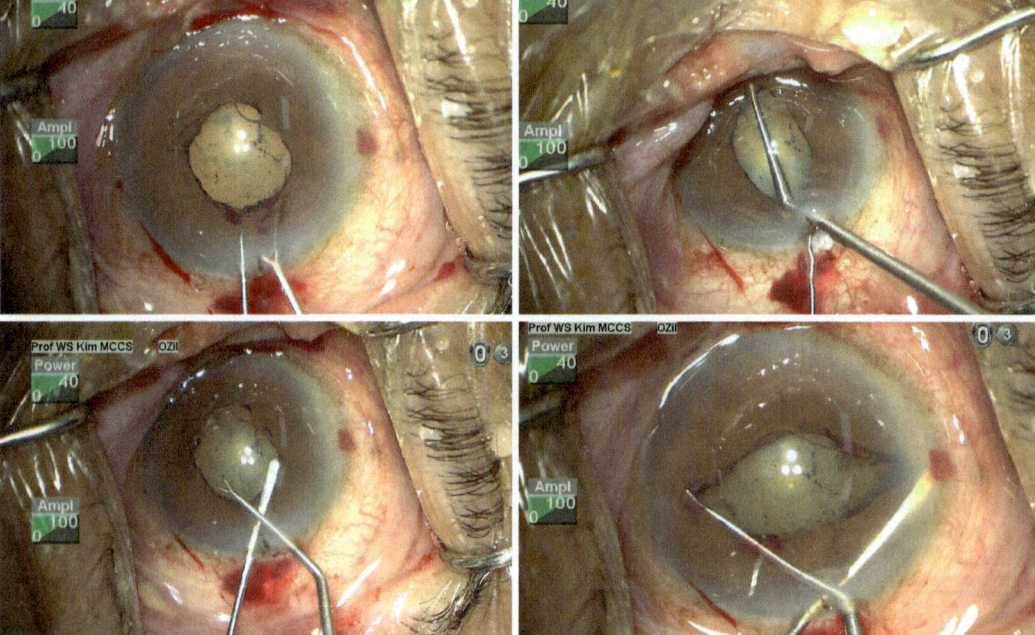

Fig. 4.5   Vertical and horizontal mechanical stretching of pupil is performed using Sinsky hook and Lens Manipulator

retraction and even during phacoemulsification due to the floppy iris.

Other Iris Dilation Using Instruments

Hydro view iris protector (Grieshaber), Morcher Pupil Expander Ring Type 5 S and Malugyn ring are being used. Each of them needs special techniques in insertion and removal of these devices.

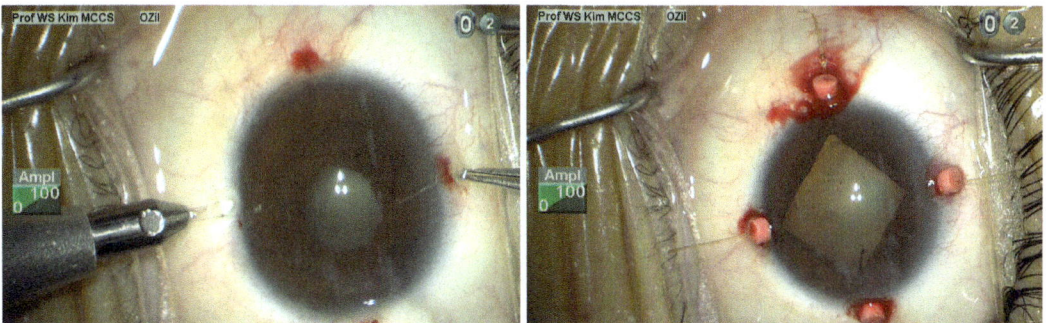

Fig. 4.6 (*Left*) Limbal paracentesis are made closer to the iris root to prevent iris pulling toward the cornea. (*Right*) Iris retractors are inserted parallel to the iris plane to dilate pupil mechanically

They cover the pupillary margin during surgery, therefore, can minimize the iris damage during surgeries. Sometimes, usage of thick instrument on the pupillary margin could disturb manipulation especially in shallow chamber, and also insertion and removal could be tricky.

Making a surgery plan in patients with cataract and glaucoma is important, because surgeons' choice of surgeries affects longevity of patients' vision. With the development of small incisional cataract surgery and antimetabolite therapy, the success of combined cataract and filtering surgery or cataract surgery alone has been improved a lot (Table 5.1).

Cataract Surgery Alone

As minimally invasive cataract surgery does not usually increase the perioperative IOP, cataract surgery alone is considered if glaucoma is adequately controlled with one or two medication and visual field loss does not involve fixation. When presence of cataract makes difficulty in visualization of optic nerve, cataract surgery is also considered. In cases with angle closure glaucoma as well as in cases with lens induced glaucoma, cataract surgery is considered alone (even without significant visual impairment), at first.

After cataract surgery alone, dangerous elevation of IOP can occur and needs more glaucoma medications.

In the presence of coexisting uveitis, excessive iris manipulation, synechiolysis, sphincterotomy, remained cortex, or remained viscoelastics will increase the risk of postoperative IOP elevation. I prefer not to use prostaglandin analogues and miotics that will increase the risk of postoperative inflammation and cystoid macular edema (CME).

Temporal incision is used to preserve superior conjunctiva for later trabeculectomy and small clear corneal incision to minimize postoperative inflammatory reaction and postoperative IOP elevation [1, 2]. Conjunctiva is spared during the surgery for the possible glaucoma filtering surgery at a later date. Glaucoma medications are continued after the surgery. IOP should be monitored carefully starting immediately after the surgery, surgeon should be readily to put additional eye drops and P.O. medications to control IOP elevations and avoid progression of visual field loss. Precautionary medications can be given immediately after the surgery for the same purpose.

Trabeculectomy Alone

Trabeculectomy alone is considered when glaucoma is not controlled with maximal glaucoma medication or unable to use glaucoma medication (due to cost, physical limitation, allergy ..) and cataract does not considered the visual threat, however, cataract will progress after glaucoma surgery. As cataract progresses after glaucoma surgery, possibility of lens-induced glaucoma should be considered. Trabeculectomy alone is performed when there is little chance to develop visually significant cataract after trabeculectomy. If cataract surgery is not feasible due to corneal edema or hyphema in cases with traumatic cataract or neovascular glaucoma, perform trabeculectomy alone and defer cataract surgery at a later date.

© Springer-Verlag Berlin Heidelberg 2016
W.S. Kim, K.H. Kim, *Challenges in Cataract Surgery*, DOI 10.1007/978-3-662-46092-4_5

Table 5.1 Indications for single or combined surgery

Operation	Indication
Phacoemulsification	A. Visually significant cataract with: 　　1. IOP well controlled with fewer than two medications 　　2. no difficulty in using available glaucoma medications 　　3. Mild-to-moderate visual field loss that does not involve or threaten fixation B. Angle closure glaucoma, and Lens induced IOP elevation
Trabeculectomy	Minimal cataract or little chance of developing visually significant cataract after trabeculectomy, with: 　　1. uncontrolled IOP with maximum tolerated medical therapy 　　2. extreme IOP elevation unless glaucoma is lens induced 　　3. unable to use medication because of cost, compliance, physical limitation, and so on
Combined Surgery	Visually significant cataract, or is likely to do so if trabeculectomy alone were performed, and: 　　1. uncontrolled IOP with maximum available medication 　　2. unable to use medications because of cost, compliance, physical limitations, and so on 　　3. extensive peripheral anterior synechia (increasing potential for postoperative IOP elevation), or mechanically blocked trabecular outflow that requires synechiolysis 　　4. visual field loss is moderate to advanced or involves fixation

Cataract surgery at the later date can result in bleb failure. I try to delay the operation as long as 1 year after trabeculectomy when the bleb becomes fully mature to prevent early bleb failure, although the incidence of bleb failure has been dramatically decreased with the introduction of antimetabolites (5-FU and MMC). However, if the development of the cataract is serious visual threat or swelling of the lens might touch the cornea, cataract surgery better be performed earlier. Surgeon should be prepared to treat failing bleb.

Cataract Surgery in the Presence of Glaucoma Filtering Bleb

Progression of cataract after filtering surgery is frequent with incidence of 15 and 42 % in our series [3, 4]. Factors related to development of glaucoma are direct trauma to lens, hypotony, flattening anterior chamber, and changes in the aqueous humor dynamics.

If the visual disturbance is not significant, it is best to wait for the cataract surgery for at least 6 months (risk of bleb failure is minimized after 1 year) [5].

The high rate of bleb failure (0–50 %) after cataract surgery in the presence of filtering bleb poses a challenge to the surgeon.

Preoperative Considerations

IOP and Bleb function needs to be evaluated before the surgery to determine the need for a trabeculectomy revision during surgery. Gonioscopy can be used to determine the patency of the sclerotomy and need for internal revision during surgery.

After glaucoma filtering surgery, it is best to delay the cataract surgery as late as possible, in order to have a mature filtering bleb that would not fail after cataract surgery. It is preferred to delay the operation more than 12 months after glaucoma filtering surgery. However, there are many occasions surgeons cannot wait that long in clinical setting. Should the surgery done before 12 month postop., precautions are needed, surgeon should be ready to deal with the failing blebs.

Large amount of postoperative astigmatism is frequently created, especially in young patients, and they should be informed about this complication before the surgery.

In advanced glaucoma patients, patients should be fully informed about the possible hazardous impact on visual outcome due to their susceptability to perioperative and postoperative IOP elevation.

Avoid any external pressure that can increase IOP before and during the surgical procedure (eg. Honan application, Peribulbar injection).

Intraoperative Considerations

Pupils are not fully dilated in many occasions, dilation performed by author is described in Chapter 4.

In glaucoma patients, manipulation of the iris including stretching of the iris (iris retractor, Malyugin ring …) should be minimized in order not to induce serious postoperative inflammation and bleb failure. Posterior surface of the iris is widely in contact with anterior surface of the anterior capsule, capsulorrhexis can be created larger than the pupil by pulling the leading edge of the capsulorrhexis towards the direction of further capsulorrhexis rather than centripetal pulling.

Location of the incision is critical, surgeon must not break the functioning bleb during the surgery, incisions must be away from the functioning bleb. I prefer to make an incisions on temporal and inferotemporal quadrant (Fig. 5.1). Even the side port incision is located away from the bleb to prevent bleb damage. Although temporal scleral incision can be an option, I prefer to make clear corneal incision that causes least postoperative inflammatory reaction and better access to the lens during surgery.

It is very important to remove all the anterior capsule fragments after capsulorrhexis, because they block the sclerotomy site if they are left in anterior chamber. To minimize postoperativeinflammatory reaction, all the nucleus and cortical material should be removed. I prefer to use acrylic foldable IOLs with PMMA haptic, because of their better anterior chamber stability.

After removal of viscoelastics, patency of the bleb can be confirmed by injecting BSS into the anterior chamber. If the bleb is not functioning, bleb revision can be performed internally using a round spatula or cyclodialysis spatula. Internal bleb revision can be performed during cataract surgery whenever the bleb is not considered functioning [3, 4].

To encourage digital massaging after surgery, corneal incision is sutured using 10–0 Nylon. Topical mitomycin was used by others and clinically proved to be effective [6, 7].

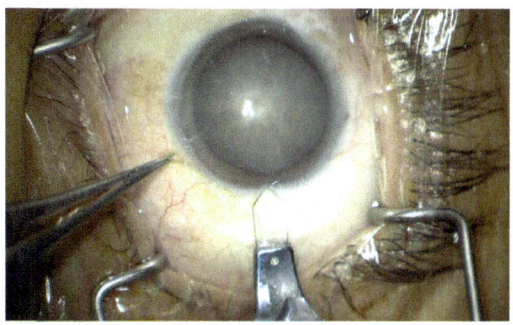

Fig. 5.1 After glaucoma filtering surgery, incisions must be away from the functioning bleb not to break the functioning bleb during surgery

Postoperative Considerations

Early postoperative IOP spikes are common, close follow up plan is required. Strict control of postoperative inflammation is the key to preserve functioning bleb. Prednisolone phosphate 1 % is given every hour while the patient is awake, then, tapers during the course of 2 months. Topical antibiotics and cycloplegics can be given.

Digital massage and 5-FU subconjunctival injection can be considered in cases with failing blebs. Since long term IOP control can be lost occasionally, close follow up is needed.

Whenever the cataract surgery is performed after glaucoma filtering surgery, surgeon should be ready to treat failing bleb. Although I try to perform cataract surgery following trabeculectomy at late as possible, not all the surgeries can wait that long or not all the patients are that much patient, surgeons are facing failing bleb not infrequently. Even eyes undergone cataract surgeries more than 12 months after glaucoma filtering surgery can develop failing bleb. All those failing bleb can be treated with FU-5 subconjunctival injection and needling procedure. Surgeons should develop their ability to deal with the failing bleb at the right timing. Patients should be aware about the possibility of failing bleb, its symptoms and consequences and should informed before the surgery about this matter.

Mainstay of the postoperative medication is strict control of postoperative inflammation and treatment of failing bleb once it happens.

Postoperative Medication

- Topical broad spectrum antibiotic: (Levofloxacin 0.5% [Cravit®, Santen, Japan] or Moxifloxacin 0.5% [Vigamox®, Alcon, USA] qid or Tobramycin 0.3% [Tobrex®, Alcon, USA] qid)
- Topical steroids: (Prednisolone acetate 1% [Pred forte®, Allergan, USA] q 1 h then tapered down to 4–8 weeks)
- Topical cycloplegics: (Tropicamide [Mydrin-P®, Santen, Japan] bid to qid or atropine sulfate 1% [Isopto atropine®, Alcon, USA] bid to qid).
- May require treatment of increased intraocular pressure: Dorzolamide/ timolol [Cosopt®, Santen, Japan] bid, Brimonidine tartrate 0.1% [Alphagan-P®, Allergan, USA] bid, Carbonic anhydrase inhibitor, acetazolamide [Acetazol®, Hanlim pharm., Korea]

Combined Cataract and Glaucoma Surgery

Standard approach for treating glaucoma and cataract together is glaucoma surgery followed by cataract surgery at a later date (3–6 months). Delay in visual recovery and expense of two surgeries, occasional failure of the filtering bleb are the drawbacks to be considered. If cataract surgery can be done at the earlier stage, it would bring the best result overall, however, progression of the glaucoma is much more urgent in many occasions.

Combined cataract and glaucoma surgeries should be considered when cataract is the main cause for visual disturbance and also the IOP is not controlled with two or more medications, other limitation to medications (allergy, cost, compliance, physical limitations…), when serious postoperative IOP rise is anticipated (extensive PAS, small atonic pupil, posterior

synechiae…), advanced visual field defect or involvement of fixation.

Options such as ciliary process photocoagulation has been reported, but it is not incorporated into our own practiced because of the less predictable effect.

With the introduction of small incision cataract surgery using foldable IOLs, a single site combined phacoemulsification with trabeculectomy has become a doable option in addition to the temporal approach clear corneal cataract extraction followed by superior trabeculectomy.

Preoperative Considerations

Preoperative evaluations include grading of cataract, status of the optic nerve, and intolerance to glaucoma medication, patients' compliance with the long term follow up. Indications for the combined surgery vary among surgeons depending on the level of experience and skill.

Antibiotic eyedrops (levofloxacin) and steroid eyedrops (prednisolone acetate 0.1%) are given every 2 h starting the day before surgery. NSAIDs (flurbiprofen sodium 0.03%) are given twice before the surgery at the day of surgery.

Topical anesthesia is given. "Pin-point" anesthesia is preferred when iris manipulation or longer surgery is expected [8]. Administration of large amount of anesthetics should be avoided.

Intraoperative Considerations

After draping, lid speculum is placed. For Fornix based incision, conjunctival limbal peritomy is made with Westcott scissors leaving the 0.5 mm of the limbal conjunctiva in order to preserve limbal germinal tissue (Fig. 5.2).

Tenonectomy is performed when patient is at high risk for bleb failure (Fig. 5.2). Hemostasis is performed using wet-field cautery. Side port inci-

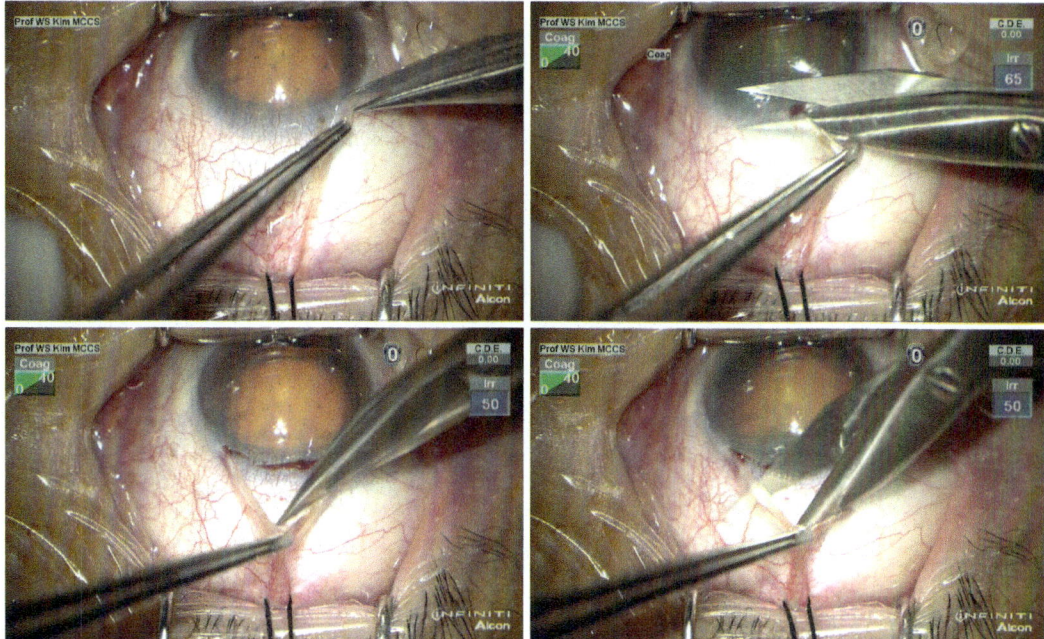

Fig. 5.2 After draping, conjunctival limbal peritomy is made with Westcott scissors. About 0.5 mm of the limbal conjunctiva should be saved to preserve limbal germinal tissue (*Top Left*, *Top Right*). Tenotomy is performed with Westcott scissors (*Bottom Left*, *Bottom Right*)

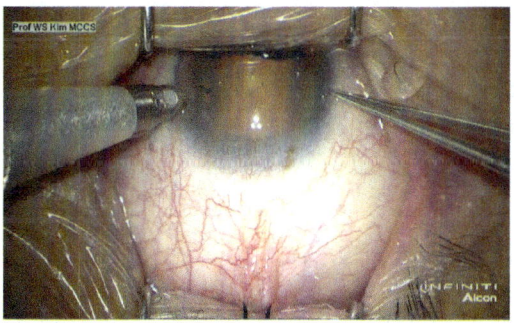

Fig. 5.3 Side port incision is made

sion is made anytime before making the main entry to the anterior chamber (Fig. 5.3).

Combined surgery can be performed using single incision or incisions can be made seperately for cataract and glaucoma surgery, their advantages are described on Table 5.2. Diamond knife or sclerotomy knife is used to fashion triangular incisions (3×3 mm) that meets at the posterior ends (Fig. 5.4). A half thickness scleral flap is made with crescent blade (Fig. 5.4). Before entering the anterior chamber, 0.2 mg/ml Mitomycin C is placed on the sclera and under the scleral flap for 3 min. Be sure not to expose the conjunctival incisional edge to Mitomycin C in order the conjunctival wound can heal without leaking during postoperative period. During all the procedures, care must be taken not to damage the conjunctival bleb by manipulating it with dressing forceps or McPherson forceps. Sac is irrigated using balanced salt solution (BSS).

Since many patients with combined glaucoma and cataract does not have reactive pupil, they should be dealt with as described in Chapter 4. After pupillary enlargement, CCC is performed using capsulorhexis forceps. I try to make 5–5.5 mm capsulorhexis (Fig. 5.5). If the CCC was not large enough to prevent capsule contraction and pupil does not dilate pharmacologically, they should be enlarged before completion of the surgery. If the pupil can be dilated pharmacologically, CCC can be enlarged using YAG laser during follow up, before capsule contraction occurs.

Table 5.2 Advantages of 1 site and 2 site phacotrabeculectomy

Procedure	Advantages
2-site phacotrabeculectomy	1. When superotemporal scarring requires superonasal filtration 2. When the presence of extremely thin conjunctiva increases the risk of a defect from the added manipulation 3. Less surgical induced astigmatism 4. Reduces postoperative scarring of the scleral flap
1-site phacotrabeculectomy	1. Don't need to change surgeon position 2. Faster than 2-site phacotrabeculectomy

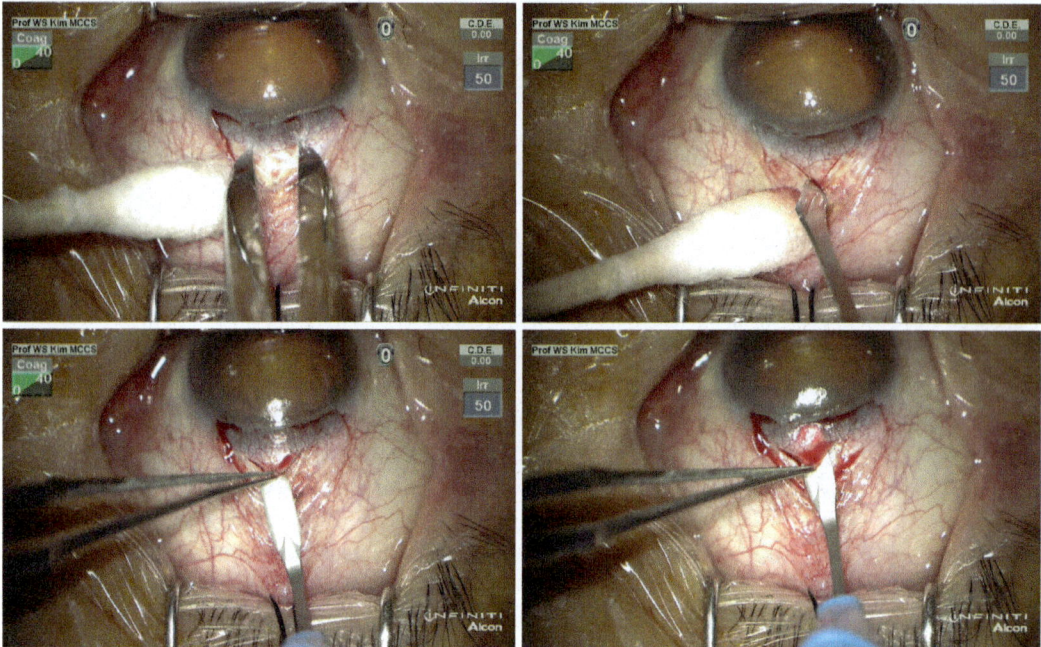

Fig. 5.4 3×3 mm triangular flap is designed and fashioned by caliper and sclerotomy knife (*Top Left, Top Right*). Half thickness scleral flap is made with crescent blade (*Bottom Left, Bottom Right*)

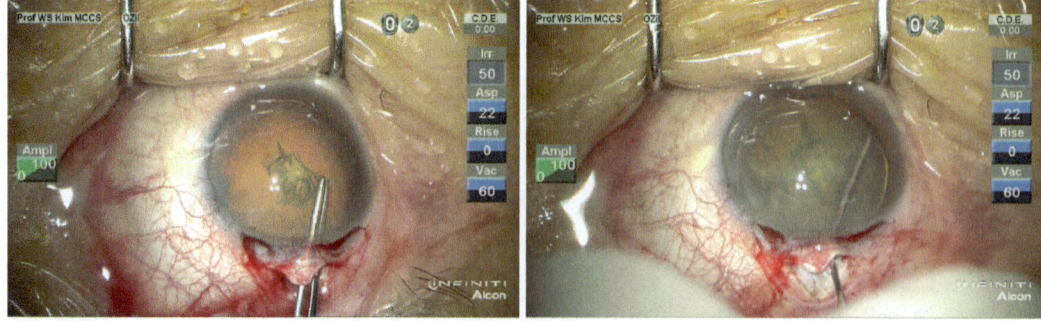

Fig. 5.5 5–5.5 mm capsulorhexis is made using capsulorhexis forceps (*Left*). Using BSS syringe, complete hydrodissection and hydrodelineation is created (*Right*)

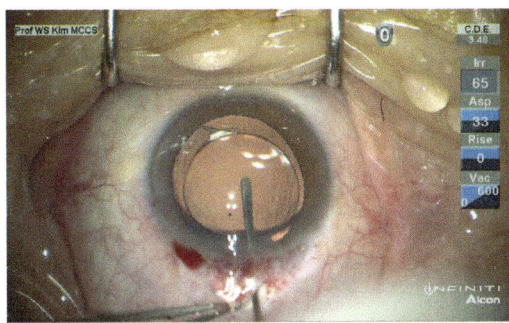

Fig. 5.6 Intraocular lens is implanted. Three-piece acrylic IOL with PMMA haptic is preferred because rigid haptic is more resistant to capsule contraction and provides more stability

Complete hydrodissection and hydrodelineation is created using BSS syringe (Fig. 5.5). Complete hydrodissection and hydrodelineation is important to facilitate the nucleus maneuverability especially when the pupils are not fully dilated.

For removal of nucleus, I prefer to use vertical chopping in cases with smaller pupil. Remove the residual cortex as clean as possible in order to minimize the postoperative inflammation, hence the secondary IOP rise.

I prefer to implant three-piece acrylic IOL with PMMA haptic for this case (Fig. 5.6). Rigid haptic is more resistant to capsule contraction, provides more stable anterior chamber, and angulated optic haptic junction prevents iridolenticular synechiae which is frequent in crowded anterior chamber or atonic pupil.

Acetylcholine (Miochol) is injected into the anterior chamber to produce miosis. A diamond knife or Crozafon punch is used to remove 1.5×1.0 mm size of trabecular meshwork (Fig. 5.7). Peripheral iridectomy is performed (Fig. 5.8). Viscoelastic is removed. Trabeclectomy flap is secured with 10–0 monofilament Nylon suture (Fig. 5.9). Placements of releasable sutures are preferred by many surgeons to control postoperative IOP elevation [9].

The conjunctiva is sutured at the limbus with 10–0 Vicryl suture (Fig. 5.10). BSS is injected to deepen the anterior chamber and inflate the bleb. The wound is checked for water tightness.

Postoperative Considerations

Rate of postop. Glaucoma filtering bleb failure is more common than that of glaucoma filtering surgery alone. Strong steroid medication is important after surgery.

Postoperative Medication

– Topical broad spectrum antibiotic: (Levofloxacin 0.5 % [Cravit®, Santen, Japan] or Moxifloxacin 0.5 % [Vigamox®, Alcon, USA] qid or Tobramycin 0.3 % [Tobrex®, Alcon, USA] qid)
– Topical steroids: (Prednisolone acetate 1 % [Pred forte®, Allergan, USA] q 1 h then tapered down to 4–8 weeks)
– Topical cycloplegics: (Tropicamide [Mydrin-P®, Santen, Japan] bid to qid or atropine sulfate 1 % [Isopto atropine®, Alcon, USA] bid to qid).
– May require treatment of increased intraocular pressure: Dorzolamide/timolol [Cosopt®, Santen, Japan] bid, Brimonidine tartrate 0.1 % [Alphagan-P®, Allergan, USA] bid, Carbonic anhydrase inhibitor, acetazolamide [Acetazol®, Hanlim pharm., Korea]

Complications

ASTIGMATISM usually more significant in young population. Amount of astigmatism is not predictable. Amount of astigmatism tends to decrease during the course of time. Glasses and contact lens correction of astigmatism may be considered.

HYPHEMA usually is self-limited.

SUBCONJUNCTIVAL HEMORRHAGE in the filtering bleb may increase the risk of bleb failure. Subconjunctival 5-FU injection can be sconsidered.

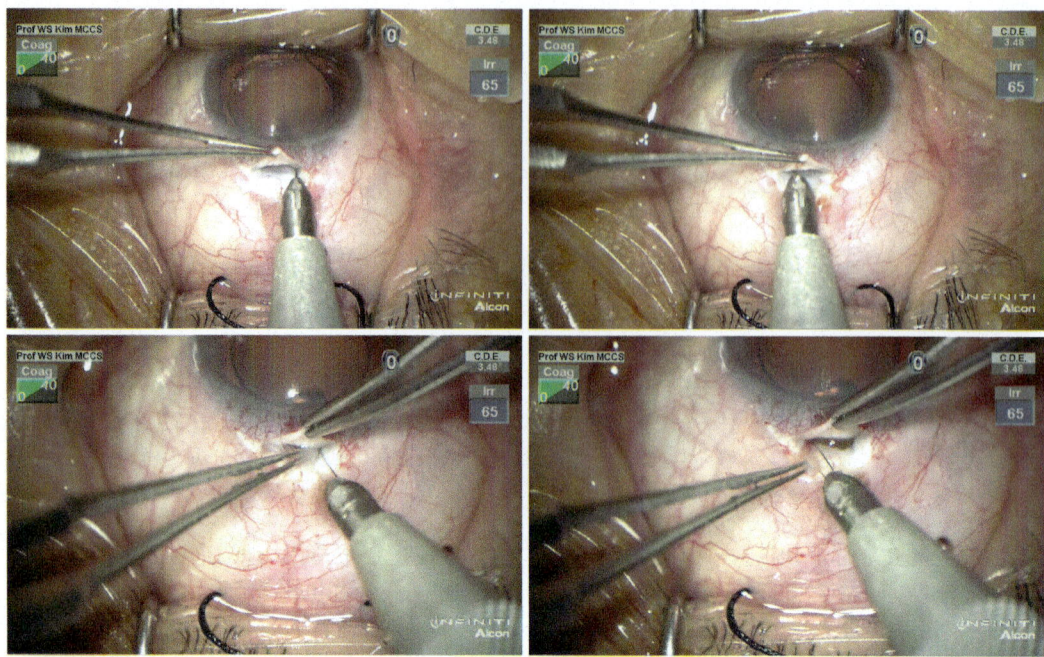

Fig. 5.7   1.5 × 1.0 mm size of trabecular meshwork is removed by diamond knife or Crozafon punch

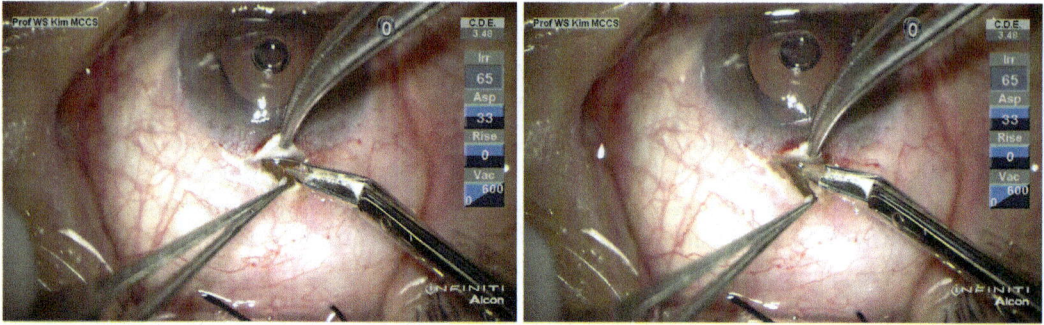

Fig. 5.8   Peripheral iridectomy is performed using iridectomy sissor

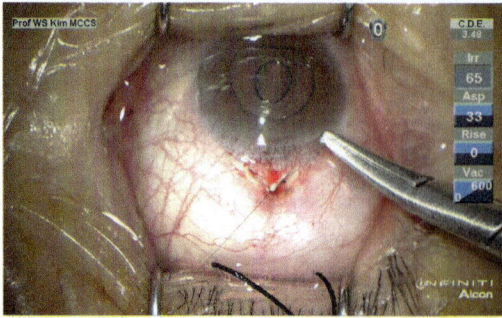

Fig. 5.9   Trabeclectomy flap is secured with 10–0 mono-filament Nylon suture

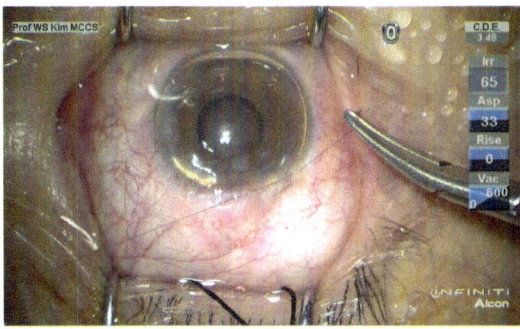 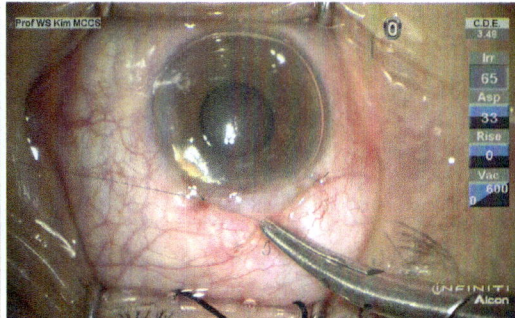

Fig. 5.10 Conjunctiva is sutured at the limbus with 10–0 Vicryl suture

CHOROIDAL DETACHMENT usually is self-limited if there's no wound leak. Cycloplegia, steroids, and use of viscoelastic can help. In cases with "kissing choroidals" immediate intervention is needed.

WOUND LEAKS are frequent. Large disposable contact lens, pressure patching over the flap, or use of cyanoacrylate glue are the treatment options for small leaks. If the leak is serious enough to make flat anterior chamber, choroidal effusion, or macular choroidal folds, intervention for should be considered.

HYPOTONUS MACULOPATHY is a more serious complication. Re-suturing of the flap must be considered.

EARLY IOP ELEVATIONS are due to remained viscoelastics, obstructed sclerotomy site by capsular fragments or tight scleral suture. When non-circulatory inflammatory cells found in the anterior chamber under slit-lamp examination, viscoelastics should be removed. Obstructed sclerotomy site is revised through surgical intervention [10]. Tight scleral suture can be released by Nd: YAG laser suturelysis [11].

LATE IOP ELEVATIONS are due to bleb failure. Bleb failure is controlled with 10 mg of 5FU injection into the bleb. Needling of bleb and scleral flap should be readily performed [12].

MALIGNANT GLAUCOMA has a symptom of shallow anterior chamber, no leak, a peripheral iridectomy and a high pressure. Cycloplegic can be sufficient in many occasions. YAG laser can be used to break the anterior hyaloid face and to redirect the aqueous flow anteriorly. However, pars plana vitrectomy is the only definitive treatment in many occasions.

BLEBITIS can occur in patients with chronic blepharitis, poor hygiene, a thin-walled bleb, an avascular bleb, and a bleb leak. Patients should be alerted to the signs and symptoms such as redness, discharge, pain, photophobia, and vision disturbance. They are treated with susceptible antibiotics.

References

1. Vu MT, Shields MB. The early postoperative pressure course in glaucoma patients following cataract surgery. Ophthalmic Surg. 1988;19:467–70.
2. Schwenn O, Dick HB, Krummenauer F, Krist R, Pfeiffer N. Intraocular pressure after small incision cataract surgery: temporal sclerocorneal versus clear corneal incision. J Cataract Refract Surg. 2001;27:421–5.
3. Seah SK, Jap A, Prata Jr JA, Baerveldt G, Lee PP, Heuer DK, Minckler DS. Cataract surgery after trabeculectomy. Ophthalmic Surg Lasers. 1996;27:587–94.
4. Crichton AC, Kirker AW. Intraocular pressure and medication control after clear corneal phacoemulsification and AcrySof posterior chamber intraocular lens implantation in patients with filtering blebs. J Glaucoma. 2001;10:38–46.
5. Cohen JS, Shaffer RN, Hetherington Jr J, Hoskins D. Revision of filtration surgery. Arch Ophthalmol. 1977;95:1612–5.
6. Cohen JS, Greff LJ, Novack GD, Wind BE. A placebo-controlled, double-masked evaluation of mitomycin C in combined glaucoma and cataract procedures. Ophthalmology. 1996;103:1934–42.
7. Budenz DL, Pyfer M, Singh K, Gordon J, Piltz-Seymour J, Keates EU. Comparison of phacotrabeculectomy with 5-fluorouracil, mitomycin-C, and without antifibrotic agents. Ophthalmic Surg Lasers. 1999;30:367–74.
8. Hansen EA, Mein CE, Mazzoli R. Ocular anesthesia for cataract surgery: a direct sub-Tenon's approach. Ophthalmic Surg. 1990;21:696–9.

9. Zhou M, Wang W, Huang W, Zhang X. Trabeculectomy with versus without releasable sutures for glaucoma: a meta-analysis of randomized controlled trials. BMC Ophthalmol. 2014;14:41.

10. Lundy DC, Sidoti P, Winarko T, Minckler D, Heuer DK. Intracameral tissue plasminogen activator after glaucoma surgery. Indications, effectiveness, and complications. Ophthalmology. 1996;103:274–82.

11. Krömer M, Nölle B, Rüfer F. Laser suture lysis after trabeculectomy with mitomycin C: analysis of suture selection. J Glaucoma. 2015;24:e84–7.

12. Ewing RH, Stamper RL. Needle revision with and without 5-fluorouracil for the treatment of failed filtering blebs. Am J Ophthalmol. 1990;110:254–9.

Posterior Polar Developmental Cataract

6

Posterior polar cataract is a large disc-shaped opacity resulting from persistent hyperplastic primary vitreous progress to degeneration of posterior subcapsular cortex and opacification. Mittendolf dot which is a remnant of a hyaloid vessel, on the posterior surface of the lens does not cause visual disturbance, however, can present thin lens capsular thickness which easily breaks during cataract surgery (Fig. 6.1).

Posterior Polar cataract is bilateral and usually inherited as autosomal dominant pattern. Cause has been suspected to be related to persistent hyaloid artery or invasion of the lens by mesoblastic tissue [1, 2].

Late developed posterior polar cataracts are usually delayed until patients feel difficulty in daily life or occupational acitivity, however, in pediatric population, close communication is necessary with pediatric ophthalmologist to balance the risk of the surgery and the risk of amblyopia when the cataract is not removed at the moment.

Preoperative Considerations

Most challenging factor when planning cataract surgery for posterior polar cataract is dealing with the posterior capsule which is very weak or even defective in posterior polar cataract.

Whorl opacity is classical but disc-shaped opacity of variable size can also be found on center of posterior capsule (Fig. 6.2).

If the lens is clear enough to visualize clumps of white flakes scattered in anterior vitreous right behind the posterior pole of the lens capsule, movement of anterior vitreous clumps gives an image of "Fish tail" movement while thea fish is moving in water ("Fish Tail Sign" by Dr. Abhay Vasavada) [3].

Opacity on capsule is frequently seen, however, is camouflaged by dense lens opacities and results in necessities vitrectomy during the course of phacoemulsification.

Visible opacificiation in subcapsular cataract is located just anterior to the posterior lens capsule secondary to steroid medications, and in association with various systemic conditions. They need to be distinguished because surgical outcome is different, and different measures must be used. Patients are informed about possible complications of the surgery, and procedures that might be given in cases with posterior capsule rupture.

Intraoperative Considerations

If longer surgery is expected, "pin-point anesthesia" is given at any stage of the operation, however, topical anesthesia is my routine anesthesia unless the patient is poorly cooperative.

© Springer-Verlag Berlin Heidelberg 2016
W.S. Kim, K.H. Kim, *Challenges in Cataract Surgery*, DOI 10.1007/978-3-662-46092-4_6

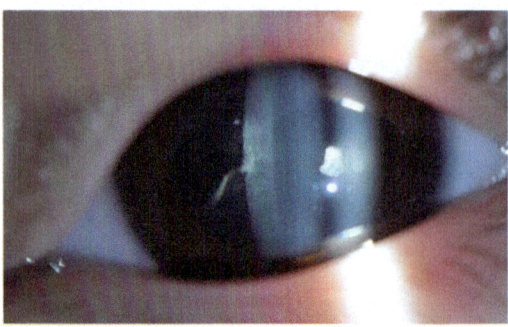

Fig. 6.1 The hyaloid vessels are present during the gestation period and regresses. If there are problems in regression, hyaloid vessel remnants can be found at slit lamp examination

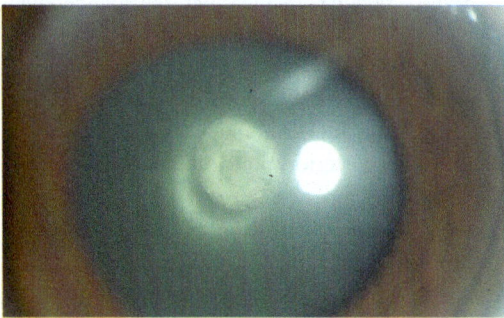

Fig. 6.2 Disc-shaped opacity can be found on posterior capsule

Keep lower bottle height throughout the surgery.

After side port incision is made, viscoelastic is injected through side port incision to maintain anterior chamber.

My preferred size of the capsulorhexis is 4–5 mm in diameter (capsular block syndrome is increased with small CCC during hydrodissection, post. Op. IOL stability is poor with large CCC in avitrectomized eye). When making a capsulrohexis in cases with possible posterior capsule rupture, surgeon needs to create a space to safely implant the IOL (sulcus placement is the next option). Hydrodelineation is needed to create s barrier between weak posterior capsule and lens nucleus during lens manipulation. I prefer to perform hydro-free hydrodissectrion using round spatula (Fig. 6.3).

Because the spatula can only separate fusion between anterior capsule and lens cortex, we can attach the posterior part of the lens cortex until later stage of the lens and cortical removal.

I try not to rotate the lens nucleus and divide the lens in situ by directing the chopper sideways. Not infrequently, the posterior epinucleus is removed during nucleus removal accidentally, lower the bottle height and "slow phaco" should be used just as we do when posterior capsule is ruptured (Fig. 6.4) [4].

For removal of epinucleus, bimanual I&A or Simcoe I&A are preferred by some surgeons for better control and better removal of the cortex. Again, maintenance of anterior chamber, avoidance of tension to posterior capsule is important until the completion of the surgery.

Before removing the instrument, viscoelastics is injected into the anterior chamber (Fig. 6.5). Even when the posterior lens capsule seems to be intact, tension to the posterior capsule should be avoided, anterior chamber and capsular bag should be properly filled with viscoelastics in order not to cause tension to the posterior capsule (if the anterior chamber and capsular bag is not properly filled with viscoelastics, vitreous pressure will push the posterior capsule forward, then posterior capsule ruptures). After IOL implantation, gentle removal of viscoelastic is needed, I try not to poke or aspirate the posterior capsule behind with I&A device in cases with posterior polar cataract even under polishing setting (vacuum 50 mmHg).

Ruptured Posterior Capsule

There are steps to take when ruptured posterior capsule is found during surgery.

1. Lower the bottle height (bottle height 50 cm) low enough not to disturb the vitreous face during insertion and removal of irrigating device (Fig. 6.6).
2. Viscoelastic injection through side port incision (I personally prefer cohesive viscoelatics

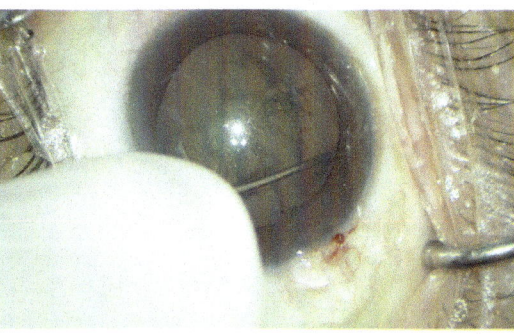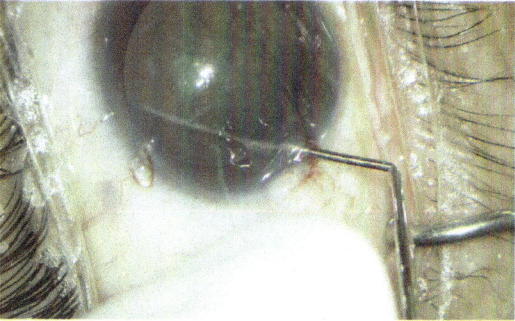

Fig. 6.3 Hydro-free hydrodissectrion is performed using round spatula to minimize posterior capsule rupture

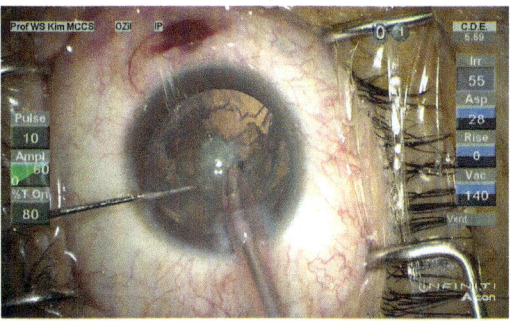

Fig. 6.4 When lens nucleus is removed "slow phaco" should be used just as we do when posterior capsule is ruptured

for easier removal at the completion of the surgery, however, dispersive viscoelastic also preferred by some surgeons because of their better visibility and chamber maintenance) (Fig. 6.6).

3. Then removal of Phaco or I&A device (If the I&A or Phaco device is removed before injection of viscoelastics, vitreous will push forward and capsular tear can be extended) (Fig. 6.6).

4. Then the ruptured edges are grasped and directed to make a rounded edge and posterior capsulorhexis. Vitrectomy is performed when dragged vitreous is found (Fig. 6.7).

IOLs are usually located in the bag, however, can be located in the sulcus when capsular sup-port is not sufficient. Capsule can be broken even during implanting soft one-piece IOL. When the capsule is broken, it starts from center of posterior capsule extends towards the equators. I prefer to transform the rupturing posterior capsule to CCC, however, posterior capsule in posterior polar cataract is usually too thin to grasp with capsulorhexis forceps, trans-formation to PCCC is not possible in many occasions. If in-the-bag IOL placement is not possible, I prefer to place one haptic in depen-dent position in the bag and another one in the sulcus, because IOL position becomes stable and permanent after capsule fusion with IOL haptic in dependent position (Fig. 6.8). The choice of IOL for this occasion should be IOLs that can be placed in sulcus with larger optic that is more acceptable in small amount of decentration (3-piece acrylic IOL with angu-lated PMMA haptic and 6–6.5 mm optic).

Postoperative Considerations

When IOL is placed in the bag with torn posterior capsule, or one haptic in the bag and one haptic in the sulcus, surgeon should warn the patient about unstable IOL and risk of IOL subluxation, their physical positioning better be restricted for 4 weeks postop. for the capsular bag to fuse together and stabilize the position of IOL permanently.

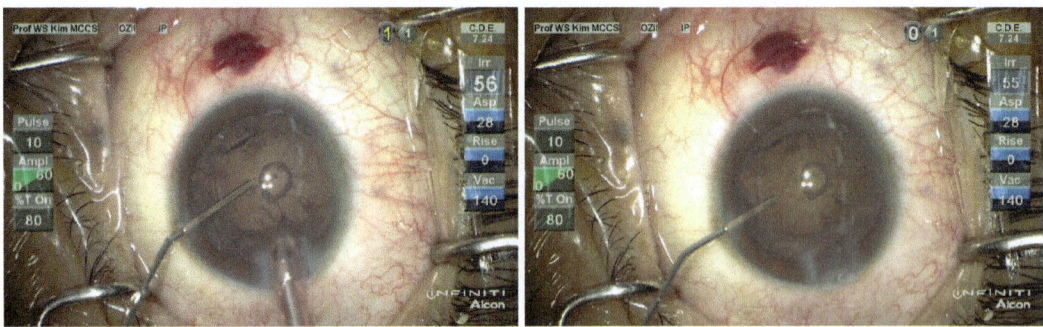

Fig. 6.5 Before removing the instrument, viscoelastics is injected into the anterior chamber to prevent posterior capsule rupture

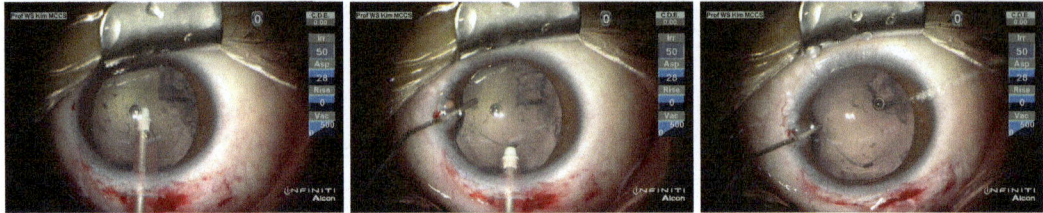

Fig. 6.6 When posterior capsule rupture is found, lower the bottle not to disturb the vitreous face during insertion and removal of irrigating device. (*Left*) Viscoelastic injection through side port incision. (*Middle*) And then remove I&A device. (*Left*)

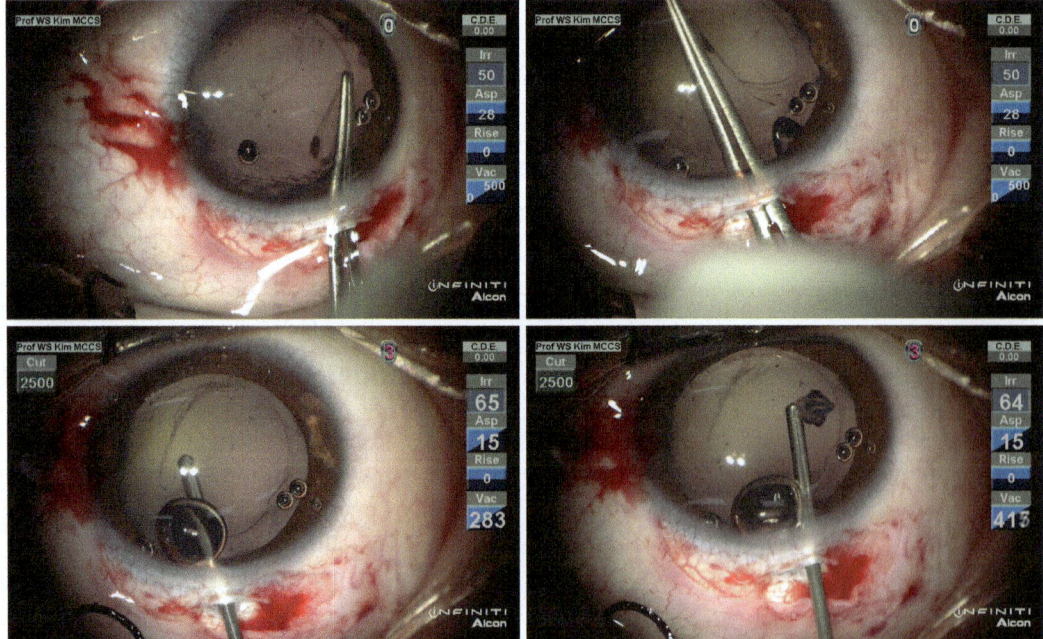

Fig. 6.7 Ruptured posterior capsule edges are grasped and posterior cpaulorhexis is made. (*Top Left, Top Right*) Anterior vitrectomy is performed to remove dragged vitreous and lens cortex. (*Middle Left, Middle Right*)

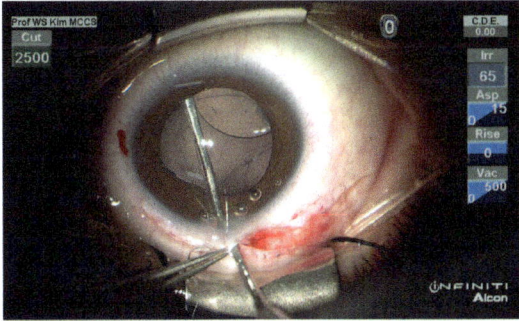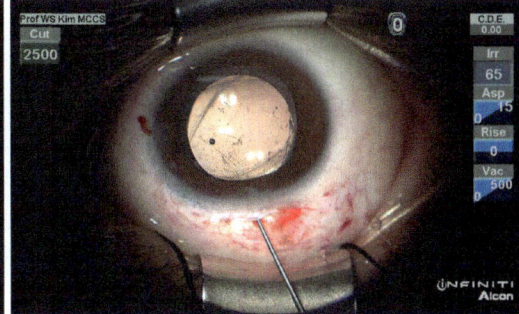

Fig. 6.8 IOL was placed one haptic in dependent position in the bag and another one in the sulcus

Postoperative Medication

– Topical broad spectrum antibiotic : (Levofloxacin 0.5 % [Cravit®, Santen, Japan] or Moxifloxacin 0.5 % [Vigamox®, Alcon, USA] qid)
– Topical steroids : (Prednisolone acetate 1 % [Pred forte®, Allergan, USA] qid)
– Topical NSAIDs : (Bromfenac [Bronuck®, Taejoon pharm., Korea] bid or Flurbiprofen sodium 0.03 % [Flurbiprofen®, Basch&Lomb, USA] qid)
– May require treatment of increased intraocular pressure: Dorzolamide/timolol [Cosopt®, Santen, Japan] bid, Brimonidine tartrate 0.1 % [Alphagan-P®, Allergan, USA] bid, Carbonic anhydrase inhibitor, acetazolamide [Acetazol®, Hanlim pharm., Korea])

References

1. Pong JC, Lai JS. Managing the hard posterior polar cataract. J Cataract Refract Surg. 2008;34:530.
2. Tulloh CG. Hereditary posterior polar cataract. Br J Ophthalmol. 1956;40:566–7.
3. Vasavada AR, Raj SM, Vasavada V, Shrivastav S. Surgical approaches to posterior polar cataract: a review. Eye. 2012;26:761–70.
4. Osher RH, Marques DM, Marques FF, Osher JM. Slow-motion phacoemulsification technique. Tech Opthal. 2003;1:75–9.

Causes of congenital cataract are most frequently idiopathic. Congenital cataract without any other systemic abnormality occurs in 1/3 of congenital cataract. Incidence of cataract caused by metabolic disease (such as galactosemia) or systemic abnormalities has been decreased due to prenatal screening.

Cataract surgery in pediatric population is much more complicated process than that of the adult population. Visual system is not completed until 8 years of age. Amblyopia is a major cause of visual impairment before and after the surgery. Surgical procedure is much more challenging especially when maneuvering the lens under soft easily distorting cornea especially when the eyes are small. Postoperative control of inflammation and close follow-up is mandatory. Incidence of complications are high, surgeons should be ready to manage the complications following the surgery.

Cataracts may develop before birth (congenital), or develop later during childhood (developmental).

Preoperative Considerations

In assessing the visual impact of the cataract, the size, density, location and patients' abnormal behavior (eg winking at day light, closing one eye…) are clues to evaluate visual impact of the cataract.

History taking from the parents is helpful in clarifying the causes of the cataract; congenital, developmental, or traumatic. And also any history of infection, maternal drug use, exposure to radiation during pregnancy should be asked. Although the number has been decreased due to the prenatal screening, there still are chances of cataracts due to metabolic condition such as galactosemia. Consult with a neonatologist will exclude every systemic conditions of the children. Even patients without any history mentioned above, patients have family history of congenital cataract not infrequently. Testing patient's urine for educing substance will exclude galactosemia and diabetes, blood calcium level can reveal neonatal tetany or infantile spasm, TORCH test can exclude some of the common infectious causes for cataracts, lens dislocation is associated with Marfan's syndrome or homocystinuria. If there's any evidence of uveitis, consult with the rheumatologies to rule out juvenile rheumatoid arthritis (JRA). In infants with congenital cataracts genetic counselling is required [1–3].

Thorough examination of both eyes of infants and young children is necessary with dilated pupil, in sedated state. Visual acuity testing in a noncompliant patient includes ability to "fix and follow", picture cards, and illiterate Es. Fundus photo is taken if possible to follow the changes in optic nerve. Refraction includes cycloplegics refraction and best corrected vision. Binocular vision function tested by pediatric ophthalmologist includes

© Springer-Verlag Berlin Heidelberg 2016
W.S. Kim, K.H. Kim, *Challenges in Cataract Surgery*, DOI 10.1007/978-3-662-46092-4_7

binocularity, fusion, stereopsis and presence of strabismus. Limitation in ocular motility, pupillary reaction including presence of afferent pupillary defect must be evaluated. Electroretinography and visual-evoked potential may be performed to evaluate neurological function of the retina and presence of amblyopia [4].

Anterior segment is examined by hand-held slit-lamp microscope to reveal lentiglobus, lenticonus, iris deformity, synechiae, zonulolysis. Size, density and extent of the cataract must be carefully examined to evaluate its impact on visual function. As the opacity is closer to the posterior pole and larger and denser, it's impact to vision is more serious. Patients' visual impact can be different among cataract patients with same size and location. Asking their behavior during daytime can be a clue to assess the impact of the cataract to the vision (If the child does not open one eye during daytime, it could cause serious amblyopia).

I prefer to consult with the pediatric ophthalmologist for impact of a certain cataract to their vision before planning cataract surgery.

Indirect ophthalmoscopy is a useful tool to reveal posterior segment abnormalities when the opacity is not dense and not total. B-scan ultrasonography is performed when visualization of the posterior segment is not feasible. Axial length measurement, corneal curvature, and IOL power calculation is attained. Intraocular pressure is measured. Corneal diameter is routinely measured in pediatric cataract to rule out microcornea or microphthlmos.

Because of its frequent association with glaucoma, gonioscopy or UBM is performed under general anesthesia.

Anatomy of the Child's Eye

Child's eyes are different from adults' eyes in size, corneal steepness, elasticity, and vitreous consistency. Most axial growth occurs during the first two years of childhood to reach mean axial length of 22 mm. Child's cornea has steep configuration. Lens is small and capsule is elastic, making the capsulorhexis challenging. Lens

substance in children is soft and the lens material and cataract is easily aspirated. Outer coat of the eye (cornea and sclera) is elastic, easily collapse during surgery especially when large incision is made.

Vitreous is more viscous and formed and attachment between anterior hyaloid face and posterior lens capsule is firm.

Variable degrees of ocular anomalies are common in congenital cataract eyes. Remnants of tunica vasculosa lentis remains in many cases. Developmental anomalies such as micophthalmia, foveal hypoplasia, optic nerve abnormalities and persistent hyperplastic accompanies.

Intraoperative Considerations

If the cataract is not considered a visual threat, frequent monitoring of the visual acuity is needed.

Timing of the Surgery

It is generally believed that visual acuity of 20/70 or less is indication for cataract surgery in pediatric cataract. Congenital monocular complete cataract should be removed within first few month (preferably 4–6 weeks of age) of life [5, 6]. I saw many patients with monocular cataract developing nystagmus and exotropia after 4 month of age, then visiting pediatric cataract surgeon. Development of strabismus or nystagmus is also an indication of surgery. Bilateral complete cataract should be removed within the first few month (preferably 6–10 weeks of age) of the surgery.

In a patient older than eight, he is not considered at risk of developing amblyopia, cataract surgery is indicated when daily activities are limited by cataract.

Usually, dense central cataract of 3 mm or larger, dense nuclear cataract, and cataract obstructing the examiner's view of the fundus are indicated for surgical removal.

Certain anterior polar, sutural, lamellar or dot cataract does not jeopardize visual function and its development and does not change with time.

These cataracts need to be followed up closely. Some doctors prefer to use cycloplegics in focal cataract to improve vision. A few patients do not tolerate photophobia and also needs glasses due to loss of accommodation.

Planing the Surgery

Before 1 years of age, lens removal without intraocular lens implantation, and use of aphakic spectacles or contact lens rehabilitation is suggested. After 1 year, an intraocular lens implantation is procedure of choice.

For binocular cataracts aged less than 1 year of age, aphakic spectacles are well tolerated. For monocular cataract aged less than 1 year of age, aphakic spectacles are not practical, large number of children would not tolerate high anisometropia, and contact lens rehabilitation is suggested.

Even in cataract patient younger than 1 year of age, amblyopic eye tends to have enlarged globe and more room for intraocular lens, and intraocular lens implantation can be performed with minimal risk for irido-lenticular synechia. However, predictability of ocular growth is poor at this age, in these eyes.

Although I prefer to implant IOL in pediatric cataract aged more than 1 year of age, implanting IOL in and eye aged less than 2 years of age is still a debate.

As ocular growth is rapid during first 2 years of life, and development of anterior segment is completed until 2 years of age, biometry measurement is reliable and ocular growth is predictable [7].

The incidence of glaucoma is high after pediatric cataract surgery. The development of glaucoma is more frequent in aphakic eyes, eyes with multiple operations, and eyes with surgery done at younger age.

In my practice, for complete bilateral cataract diagnosed at birth, I perform cataract removal, anterior & posterior capsulorhexis, and anterior vitrectomy 1 week apart as soon as possible, no later than 4 month of age. Secondary implantation of IOL is usually after 2 years' of age, or

contact lens intolerance. Now, I prefer to delay the secondary implantation of the IOL because incidence of glaucoma drops rapidly as the child grows. Parents of the children want to implant the IOL before school age, surgeon need to discuss these matters with parents seriously.

For complete monocular cataract, surgery should be done as soon as possible, and implantation of the IOL is routinely considered after 1 years of age, or amblyopic cataractous eye is larger than sound eye and is considered to have room for IOL placement. If IOL is not implanted, contact lens is used for visual rehabilitation. For contact lens is used for visual rehabilitation after surgery for young children, contact lenses are thick and easily lost, parents should be attentive to the child, and should inform the doctor when the child resists to the contact lens to consider secondary IOL implantation.

Lens Removal, PCCC, and Anterior Vitrectomy (Cataract Aged Less Than 1 Year of Age)

Surgery is performed under general anesthesia. Children's pupils are not readily reactive to mydriatics. However, use of too much phenylephrine can cause elevated blood pressure and irritable myocardium. In many occasions, examinations including biometry is not accurate at out-patient clinic, repeated biometry including keratometry, refraction, and intraocular pressure measurement is needed. For this purpose, many portable instruments are needed. Keratometry is measured by Retinomax K-Plus 3 (Right Med, Virginia Beach, VA). For careful observation hand held slitlamp can be used. As glaucoma is accompanied in 25–31 % of patients in pediatric cataract patient, Tono-Pen AVIA tonometer (Reichert Inc, Buffalo, NY), Icare-Pro tonometer (Icare, Tiolat Oy, Helsinki, Finland) and Perkins applanation tonometry (Perkins; Clement-Clarke, Haag-Streit, UK) are used for IOP measurement. IOP is measured preoperatively and postoperatively at each visit.

Superior bridle suture is made at superior rectus muscle, however, this is for rotation of the globe inferiorly when suture is placed on superior incision at the completion of the surgery (Fig. 7.1). For better visualization of the capsule during anterior and posterior capsulorhexis, globe is placed coaxial to the illumination.

Paracentesis incision is made on 2–3 o'clock position on limbus. For elastic corneas in younger population, tunnel should be longer than usual or suture may be needed at the completion at the surgery to prevent leaking. Before making a main incision, viscoelastic is injected into the anterior chamber.

As corneal incision can create large amount of astigmatism after cataract surgery in young children with soft cornea and sclera, I prefer to make superior scleral incision 2 mm behind the limbus 2.2 mm in width (Fig. 7.2).

Capsulorhexis is performed with cystotome, bent needle, or capsulorhexis forceps (Fig. 7.3). For elastic pediatric capsule, firm pressure is needed to create a central puncture. Capsulorhexis forceps are used to grasp and guide the tear radially until it reaches a desired diameter, then direct the capsulorhexis parallel to the pupillary margin. During capsulorhexis, in order not to make radial tear in elastic pediatirc capsule, capsule

staining can be used to decrease the elasticity; viscoadaptive viscoelastic use can minimize the tension exerted on lens capsule by decreasing the expansion of the capsule. Viscoelastic is used until the capsular tension is minimum. If too much viscoelastic is used, capsule will be pushed backward behind the zonular attachment, capsular tension will be increased again. When injecting Viscoelastics, it is injected on the capsule which is about to be torn because we need to decrease the tension on the capsule on that quadrant. Because of its tendency of radial extension, frequent regrasping and frequent use of high viscosity viscoelastics are useful for successful capsulorhexis.

Some doctors prefer to use vitrectorrhexis, radio-frequency diathermy, and can be used is too elastic cases, however, their edge margin are not as resistant as capsulorhexis margin to tear.

Most nuclei are soft, there's no need to use phacoemulsification. Coaxial and bimanual irrigation–aspiration device use is needed to meticulously remove all the cortex (Fig. 7.3).

Posterior capsulorhexis is made to capture the IOL and then prevent development of after cataract. In our study, optic capture technique

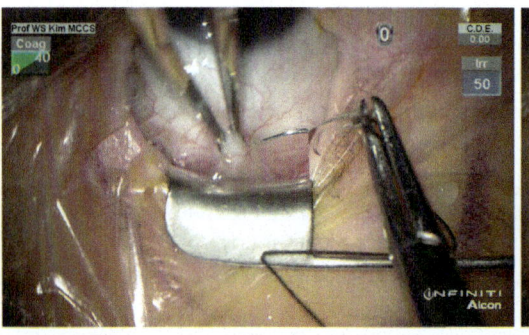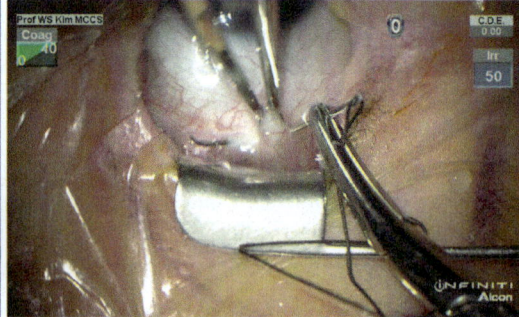

Fig. 7.1 Superior bridle suture is made at superior rectus muscle

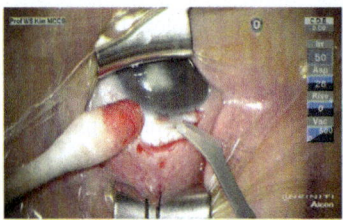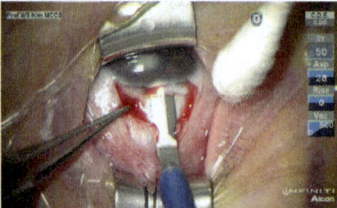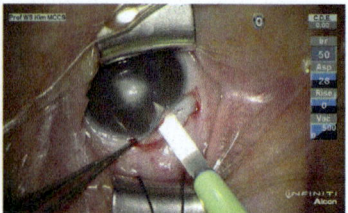

Fig. 7.2 Superior scleral incision is made at 2 mm behind the limbus 2.2 mm in width

also decrease the development of glaucoma after surgery [8].

After aspiration of the lens cortex, anterior chamber is filled with viscoelastics, capsular bag should not be distended with viscoelastics (Fig. 7.4).

A 26-gauge bent needle make a central puncture by firm pressure on posterior capsule. Try to lift up the torn capsule leaflet upward to have a better grasp with the forceps. Viscoelastic can be injected though the puncture to separate the central 4–5 mm diameter circle of anterior vitreous face to posterior capsule. Using capsulorhexis forceps, posterior capsulorhexis (PCCC) is created as CCC, with a size of 3.5–4 mm in diameter (Fig. 7.4). Be sure to keep in mind that PCCC should be small than ACCC. If PCCC is larger than ACCC, surgeon would have difficulty implanting the IOL in the bag, IOL will keep falling into the vitreous cavity. Importance of manual PCCC is that it ensures resistance to radial tear during vitrectomy (when IOL is not implanted during first surgery) and also during optic capturing procedure (when IOL is implanted during first surgery).

If capsule is torn during ACCC or PCCC, it should be described in the record in order to make a right implantation plan for the secondary IOL implantation surgery.

Anterior Vitrectomy should be performed when IOL is not implanted. As the vitreous in small children are highly reactive, if vitreous face is in continuity with capsulorhexis margin, thick fibrous opacities will occur. It is because of the scaffolding of the vitreous face to the migrating and proliferating lens epithelial cells. Vitrectomy is performed until the continuity of the capsulorhexis margin to the anterior vitreous is lost (Fig. 7.4). IF the continuity is lost between vitreous and capsulorhexis, vitrectomy cutter placed under the capsulorhexis margin does not pull the PCCC margin during cutting procedure in 360°. Vitrectomy cutter placed under the CCC margin is performing vitrectomy with the cutter opening facing upward and keep a space between the cutter and the capsule. High-speed cutting is needed in order not to damage the integrity of PCCC and not to drag the retina. It is also important to move the cutter slowly sideways to allow the cutter tip to clear the vitreous around. During vitrectomy if any vitreous strand is noticed, vitrectomy should be performed while approaching to the vitreous strand, rather than leaving the vitreous strand. At least two incisions are used for entry of vitrectomy cutter to ensure removal of vitreous under the PCCC thoroughly.

In small children, removal of anterior 1/3 of the vitreous is adequate by most of the pediatric cataract surgeons. I try to remove the vitreous behind the posterior capsule until the vitrectomy cutter placed behind CCC margin does not drag the fringe of the PCCC.

Placement of intraocular lens in a child younger than 1 year of age is technically challenging and causes a lot of unpredictable complications.

All the incisions including scleral and side port incisions should be inspected for need for closure. Main incisions are always closed using 10–0 nylon, or 9–0 Vicryl because children tend to rub the eyeball. Side port incision, also are frequently closed with same material. If large incision was made (6–6.5 mm) internal portion of the wound should be checked for gaping using

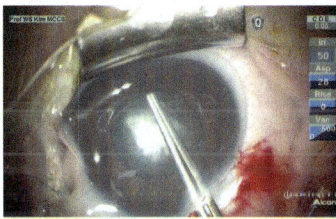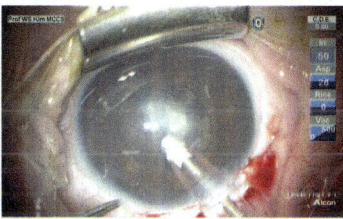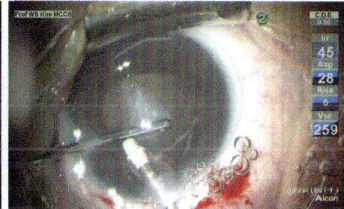

Fig. 7.3 Capsulorhexis is performed with capsulorhexis forceps. (*Left*) Coaxial and bimanual I&A is used to removed lens nucleus and cortex. (*Middle*, *Right*)

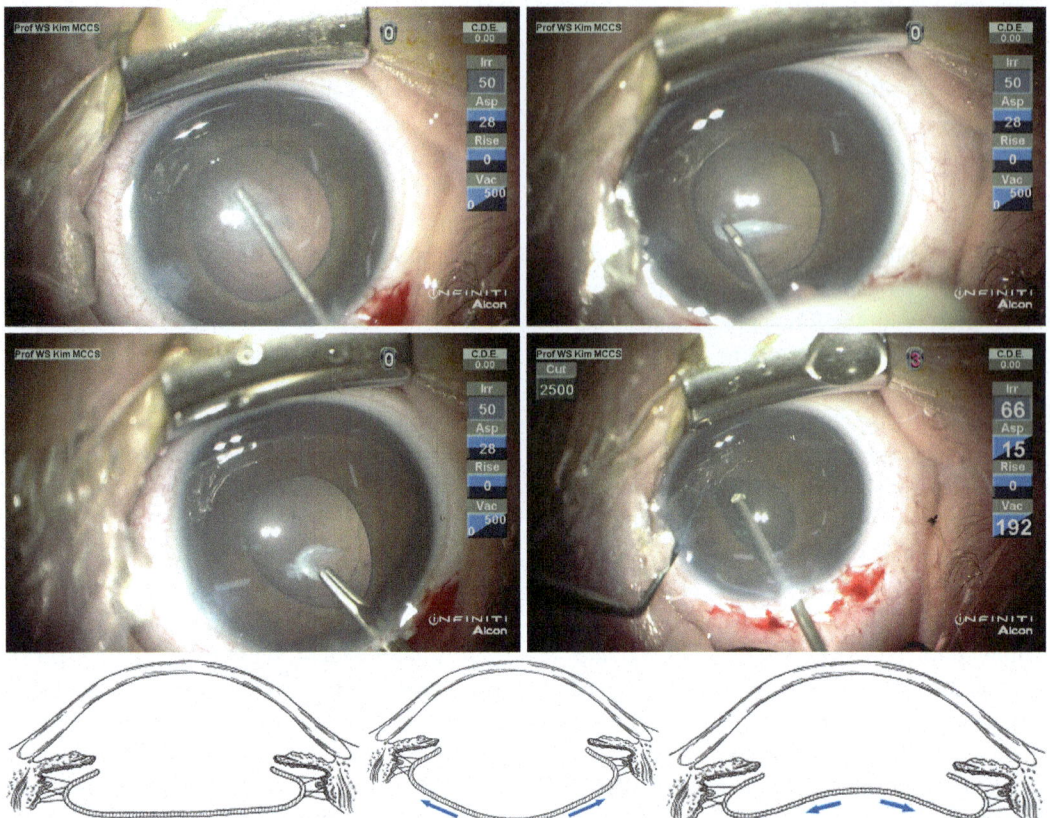

Fig. 7.4 Anterior chamber is filled with viscoelastics, capsular bag should not be distended with viscoelastics. (*Top Left*) Too much or too less viscoelastics can cause capsular tensions. (*Bottom Left*, *Bottom Middle*, *Bottom Right*) Using bent needle and capsulorhexis forceps, pos-terior capsulorhexis is created, with a size of 3.5–4 mm in diameter. (*Top Right*, *Middle Left*) Vitrectomy is per-formed until the continuity of the capsulorhexis margin to the anterior vitreous is lost. (*Middle Right*)

gonioscopy mirror. 10–0 nylon full thickness suture for internal gaping is needed if any gap is found. Flared margin can also be closed when injecting air into the anterior chamber.

Lens Removal and IOL Implantation (Cataract Aged More Than 1 Year of Age)

Lens implantation is indicated in cataract in pat-ents older than 1 year of age [9, 10]. Biometry is fairly predictable after 2 years of age. In monocu-lar cataract, and in contact lens intolerant patent, IOL implantation can be considered at earlier.

I prefer to use foldable three-piece acrylic biconvex IOL with large optic (6–6.5 mm in diameter) and PMMA haptic, overall length between 12.5 and 13.5 mm. Haptics are C loop or J loop (preferably modified C loop). Foldable IOL allows creation of small incisions that do not produce large amount of post-operative astigma-tism. Among foldable IOLs, acrylic IOL is more controllable during implantation, and produces minimal inflammation. Large sized IOL optic provides larger area of optical correction, and is more forgiving to some amount of decentration within the capsular bag. Surface modified lens could have an advantage. Rigid haptic can pre-vent capsular contraction that can easily occur after pediatric cataract. Haptic angulation mini-mizes the IOL's contact with the iris, thus the synechia. PMMA haptic three-piece IOL is used for IOL optic capturing to the posterior capsule.

Table 7.1 IOL power selection

Ages	Target refraction
12 months	+7–8
2 year	+5
3 year	+4
4 year	+3
5 year	+2

Power selection of IOL should be considered according to the age of patients (Table 7.1).

When optic capturing is not used, single piece acrylic IOLs are preferred by many surgeons. Certain single piece acrylic IOL has easier to implant through small incision, superior memory function and good centration.

There have been many attempts to use multi-focal IOLs in pediatric cataract. Their potential benefits are compensation for presbyopia, greater spectacle independence, however, centration will change with growth, in accurate biometry in child's eye, change in astigmatism and refraction during growth, amblyopiogenic effect of multiple images focused on retina, decreased contrast sensitivity, photic phenomenon will impede the development of better vision of developing visual system. I personally discourage using multifocal IOLs in children who's visual system is still developing. Because of their poorer optical quality does not guarantee best corrected vision, continuously growing children's eye, refractive status of the growing children's eye continuously changing, and multiple images focusing macula could be confusing and amblyopiogenic.

IOL Optic Capturing to Posterior Capsule

I prefer to use foldable three-piece acrylic biconvex IOL with large optic (6–6.5 mm in diameter) and PMMA haptic, overall length between 12.5 and 13.5 mm. Haptics are C loop or J loop (preferably modified C loop). Foldable IOL allows creation of small incisions that do not produce large amount of post-operative astigmatism. Among foldable IOLs, acrylic IOL is more controllable during implantation, and

produces minimal inflammation. Large sized IOL optic provides larger area of optical correction, and is more forgiving to some amount of decentration within the capsular bag. Surface modified lens could have an advantage. Rigid haptic can prevent capsular contraction that can easily occur after pediatric cataract. Haptic angulation minimizes the IOL's contact with the iris, hence the synechia. PMMA haptic three-piece IOL is used for IOL optic capturing to the posterior capsule.

Single-piece acrylic IOL is not a lens for posterior capsule capture of IOL optic. Their thickness of optic-haptic junction does not allow optic capture and softness of the material bend the optic haptic junction when captured to the posterior capsule.

Capsulorhexis, I&A and PCCC are performed as described previously. Anterior vitrectomy may or may not be performed. Optic capture techniques, which I believe is the best way to preserve clear visual axis, was introduced by Dr. Gimbel.

Posterior capsule capturing of the IOL optic is carried out under the presence of viscoelastic filled anterior chamber. Suture may or may not be placed to the main incision. Using round spatula IOL optic 90° away from the IOL haptic junction is slipped though the PCCC margin on one side. Then, same procedure is done on the other side of the IOL optic (Fig. 7.5). It is important to make a tight capturing of the IOL optic, to have permanent capturing, and to have complete compartmentalization of the anterior vitreous face, which is hyperactive to inflammatory cells. If capturing is loose, inflammation in anterior chamber will propagate towards anterior vitreous face, chances of vitreous face opacification will increase. Usual target size for PCCC is the diameter 1.5 mm smaller than the implanting IOL optic, however, posterior capsules of lenticonus and lentiglobus are too thin to create a properly sized capsulorhexis. Thin capsules, younger capsules are more elastic, and expands larger degree than older ones.

Viscoleastic is removed with I & A device or by injecting BSS into the anterior chamber. With use of cohesive viscoelastics, viscoelastic can be

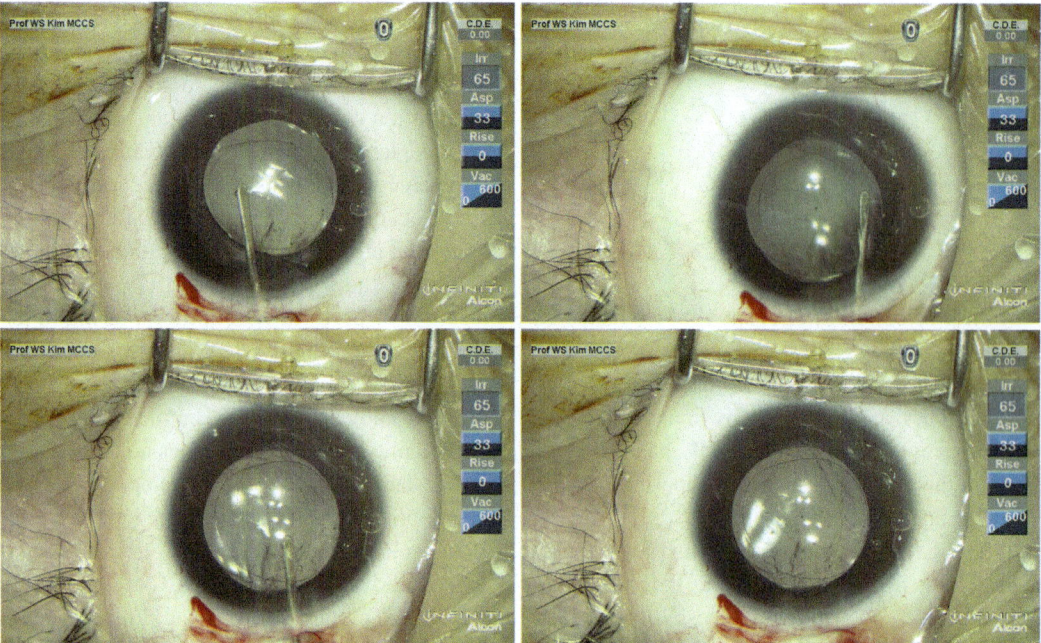

Fig. 7.5 IOL optic 90° away from the IOL haptic junction is slipped though the PCCC margin on one side. (*Top Left, Top Right*) Same procedure is done on the other side of the IOL optic. (*Bottom Left, Bottom Right*)

removed through side post incision or through main incision between suture bites by elevation of pressure with BSS.

There were occasions when peripheral tear was created in the posterior capsule during IOL optic capturing:

1. If the IOL is captured and stable when the tear is found on one side, leave the IOL, close the wound, and remove the viscoelastic without fluctuation of anterior chamber. The capsule will fuse to form a stable captured IOL-capsule complex.
2. If the bag integrity is lost, IOL is not stable in the bag, pull the IOL optic anteriorly through CCC to make anterior capsule capturing of IOL.
3. If the bag integrity is lost, IOL is not stable, anterior capsule capturing of IOL cannot be performed due to poor sizing, IOL is relocated to sulcus, by dial the lens using Sinsky hook.

In spite of these technical difficulties, I try to perform posterior capsule capture of IOL optics whenever possible, because it prevents development of after cataract, decrease postoperative inflammation,

and decrease development of glaucoma [8]. There are occasions when optic capturing cannot be performed; posterior capsular tear, extremely decentered PCCC, too large PCCC. In cases with capsular plaque that extends to far periphery, and proper sizing of capsulorrhexis is often challenging.

Wound closure and medication is given as described previously.

Pars Plana Vitrectomy

I believe pars plana rarely indicated and performed in cases with microcornea, microphthalmia or small pupil. Its advantages are reduced incidence of vitreous incarceration, retinal traction and detachment after surgery, easier access to lens periphery, and less damage to corneal endothelium. However, this technique loses capsular bag integrity, limits safety of IOL placement, decreases options for optical rehabilitation. Child's pars plana is still developing, complications such as retinal dialysis and ciliary body detachment can occur not infrequently.

I prefer to use limbal vitrectomy if vitrectomy is necessary.

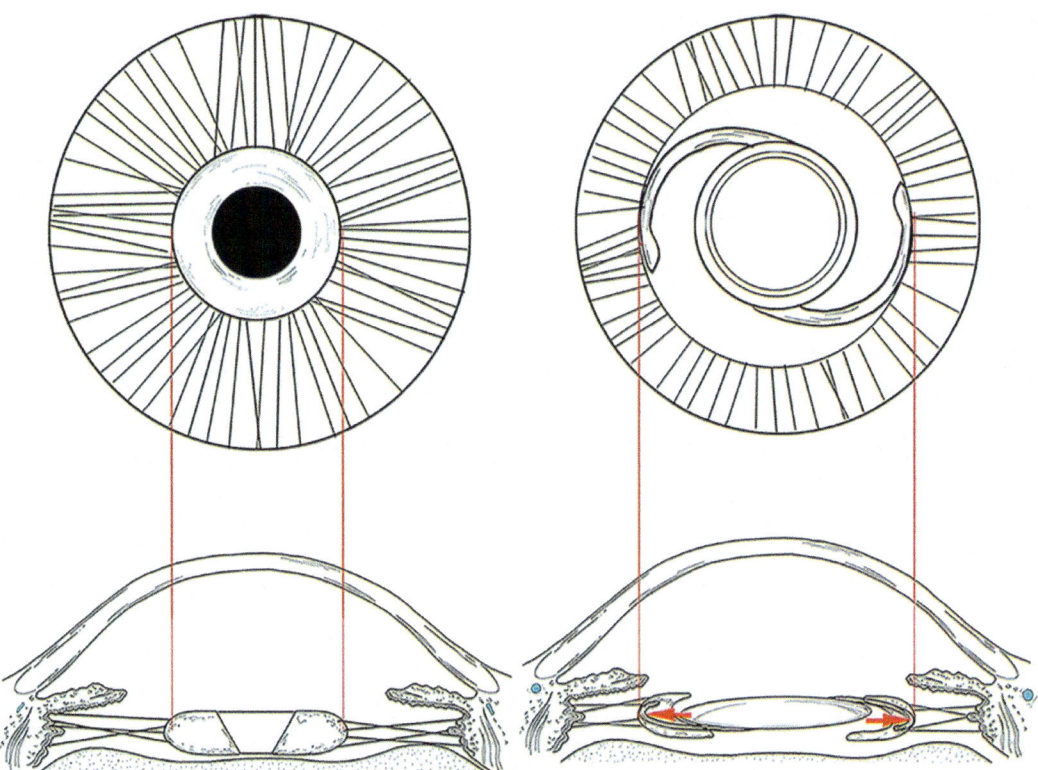

Fig. 7.6 Fused capsular bag contracts and pulls the 360° of ciliary body inwards, distorts aqueous outflow channel. (*Left*) By relieving this contraction with in the bag IOL implantation, aqueous flow can be improved by facilitation of aqueous drainage (*Right*)

Secondary IOL Implantation in Children

I prefer to implant secondary implantation of the IOL when the child reaches age of two when biometry of the children becomes as predictable as that of the adults. However, if aphakic children's eye develop glaucoma and become not controllable with glaucoma medication, I implant PC IOL with PMMA haptic in the bag. In my case series, most glaucoma could be treated or medically controllable. I hypothesize that, as children grows, fused capsular bag contracts and pulls the 360° of ciliary body inwards, distorts aqueous outflow channel. By relieving this contraction with in the bag IOL implantation, aqueous flow can be improved by facilitation of aqueous drainage (Fig. 7.6).

When aphakic patients came in to the office, we need to dilate the pupil, and inspect the integrity of the lens capsule. In many cases, pupils do not

dilate well. If the previous surgery was performed at the same clinic or a well-documented operation record is given, surgeon can plan where the IOL can be placed. If the patients posterior capsule was torn at previous surgery, IOL should be placed in the sulcus in front of the Sommering ring.

First, 1 mm side port incision is made on 2–3 o'clock position. Viscoelastic is introduced into the anterior chamber. Main incision is made on superior quadrant in 2.2 mm in size.

Viscoelastic cannula and round spatula is used to remove adhesions between capsular leaflet and back surface of the iris (Fig. 7.7). If iridectomy is present on superior quadrant, instrument can be passed through iridectomy.

After removal of all the adhesions, iris is retracted with manipulator 360° for inspection of integrity of the remaining capsule. If previous surgery was completed as planned, viscoelastic cannula and round spatula is used to open fused anterior and posterior capsular leaflet (Fig. 7.8).

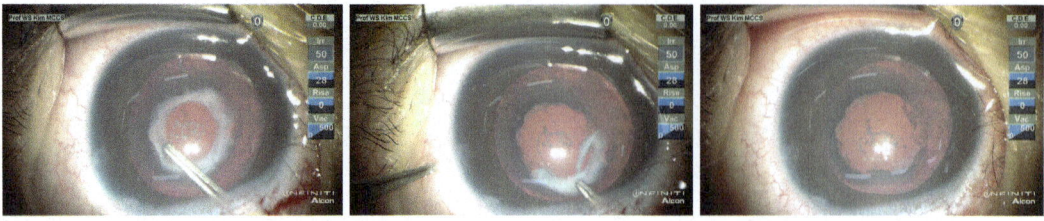

Fig. 7.7 Viscoelastic cannula and round spatula is used to remove adhesions between capsular leaflets

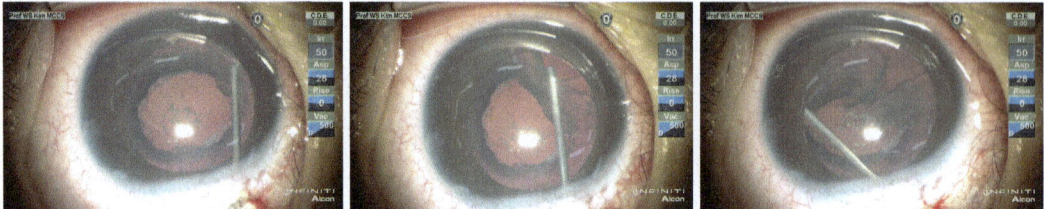

Fig. 7.8 Viscoelastic is used to open fused anterior and posterior capsular leaflet and viscodissect cortical material

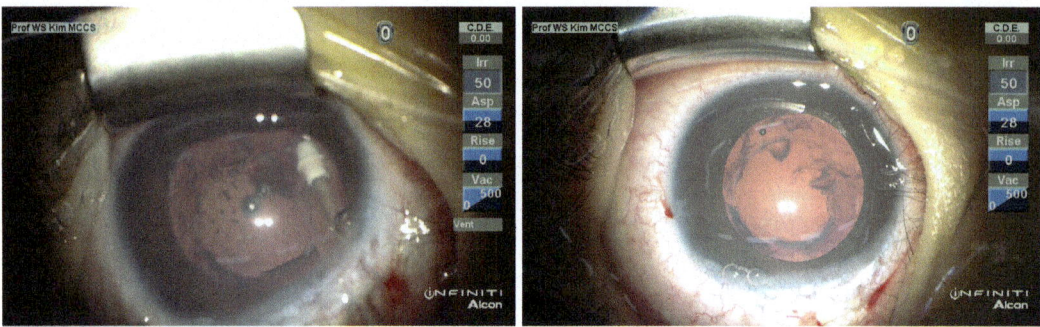

Fig. 7.9 Cortical material is removed using I&A device at low bottle height

Cortical material is removed using I&A device at low bottle height (Fig. 7.9).

Leading haptic of the implanting IOL is placed into the capsular bag of 6 o'clock position (Fig. 7.10). Placement of the leading haptic is important. To place the IOL in the bag easily, PCCC should have been made smaller than ACCC. In cases with large PCCC, retraction of CCC on 6 o'clock position can be needed. If IOL's leading haptic is placed in the bag, IOL is dialed into the capsular bag.

Wound closure is performed as described previously.

There are doctors implanting IOL in the bag without posterior capsulorhexis. After cataract will develop in 100 % of the cases. If the patient is cooperative enough, Nd-YAG laser capsulotomy can be performed at a later date. In many occasions, if the patient is not cooperative enough, IOL damage can occur due to poorly focused Nd-YAG laser. IOL damage can occur due to high-powered laser, which is frequently needed to break thick fibrosed posterior capsule. Another finding is children's vitreous gel, which is attached to the posterior capsule and does not fall down in the vitreous cavity.

Worst scenario would be implanting IOL in the bag with posterior capsulorhexis but without vitrectomy, vitreous will fuse to form thick fibrosed plaque of vitreous face and posterior capsule.

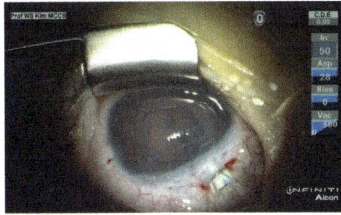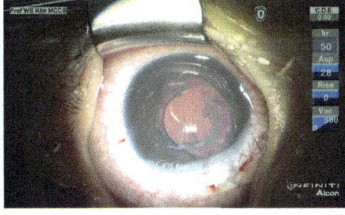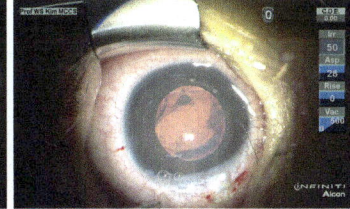

Fig. 7.10 After leading haptic of the implanting IOL is placed into the capsular bag of 6 o'clock position, trailing haptic is also rotated towards the capsular bag

Postoperative Considerations

Strict control of post-operative inflammation and prevention of complications caused by inflammation is the mainstay in post-operative mediations. Refraction correction and amblyopia treatment is given within 1 week after surgery and continues until the visual system gets mature.

IOP is checked on every visit (POD1/POD3/1st week/2nd week/4th week/8th week/12th week/ then every 2 months until the end of 1 year).

Fundus photography is taken for follow up of optic disc change and fundus using hand-held fundus camera.

Before discharging from the hospital patient is sent to the pediatric ophthalmologist for amblyopia treatment plan and glasses prescription. Whatever refractive error children might have after surgery, they are not going to stable over time. They should be frequently followed until they develop fully mature vision.

Postoperative Medication

– Topical broad spectrum antibiotic: (Tobramycin 0.3 % [Tobrex®, Alcon, USA] qid)
– Topical steroids: (Prednisolone acetate 1 % [Pred forte®, Allergan, USA] q 1 h then tapered down to 4–8 weeks)
– Topical cycloplegics: (Tropicamide [Mydrin-P®, Santen, Japan] q 10 min 6 times and atropine sulfate 1 % [Isopto atropine®, Alcon, USA] qid for 2–4 weeks to continuously move the pupil then prevent synechiae formation).

– Topical NSAIDs: (Bromfenac [Bronuck®, Taejoon pharm., Korea] bid or Flurbiprofen sodium 0.03 % [Flurbiprofen®, Basch&Lomb, USA] qid)
– May require treatment of increased intraocular pressure: Dorzolamide/timolol [Cosopt®, Santen, Japan] bid, Brimonidine tartrate 0.1 % [Alphagan-P®, Allergan, USA] bid, Carbonic anhydrase inhibitor, acetazolamide [Acetazol®, Hanlim pharm., Korea]

References

1. Zetterström C, Lundvall A, Kugelberg M. Cataracts in children. J Cataract Refract Surg. 2005;31:824–40.
2. Nelson LB. Diagnosis and management of cataracts in infancy and childhood. Ophthalmic Surg. 1984;15:688–97.
3. Del Monte MA. Diagnosis and management of congenital and developmental cataracts. Ophthalmol Clin North Am. 1990;3:205–19.
4. Ohzeki T. The value of electro-physiological testing in assessment of visual function in children. Eur J Implant Refract Surg. 1990;2:249–52.
5. Stark WJ, Taylor HR, Michels RG, Maumenee AE. Management of congenital cataracts. Ophthalmology. 1979;86:1571–8.
6. Gelbart SS, Hoyt CS, Jastrebski G, Marg E. Long-term visual results in bilateral congenital cataracts. Am J Ophthalmol. 1982;93:615–21.
7. van Balen AT, Koole FD. Lens implantation in children. Ophthalmic Paediatr Genet. 1988;9:121–5.
8. Lee CK, Kim SS, Kim WS. Glaucoma following pediatric cataract surgery: incidence and risk factors. J Korean Ophthalmol Soc. 2011;52:1150–60.
9. Binkhorst CD, Gobin MH. Congenital cataract and lens implantation. Ophthalmologica. 1972;164:392–7.
10. Gimbel HV, Ferensowicz M, Raanan M, DeLuca M. Implantation in children. J Pediatr Ophthalmol Strabismus. 1993;30:69–79.

Cataract Surgery in Eyes with Trauma

8

Ocular trauma is frequently associated with cataractous changes in the lens in up to 60% of patients, and crystalline lens damage is present in 30% of perforating injuries of the anterior segment of the eye [1]. Traumatic cataract can occur due to penetrating ocular trauma, or may also result from blunt injury. Their extent and nature of the injuries are difficult to assess accurately. Frequently accompanying lesions are, corneal laceration, scleral laceration, accompanying iris incarceration, iris dialysis, tear or laceration of iris, hyphema, vitreous herniation, lens subluxation or dislocation into anterior chamber or posteriorly into vitreous cavity. The level of involvement of the anterior and posterior segment, visibility of internal structure, availability of materials or instruments being used for expected anterior or posterior segment procedure, materials for surgical repair, and possible scenarios expected with given information should be dully considered. Before surgery, patient counseling is important, they should be warned about the worst scenarios expected after the surgery. And also, should be informed about possibility of multiple surgeries.

Preoperative Considerations

The level of surgical technique required for traumatic cataract is high. The accompanied injuries on various structures must be assessed, however, the initial assessments are not always enough or accurate, many complicated situations can be found during operation. Careful history taking is mandatory to evaluate the nature of the injury (open or closed, presence of posterior segment trauma, or presence of IOF) how the injury has occurred.

Preoperatively, precisely assess the extent and degree of ocular damage, set up operation plan, and prepare all instruments potentially in need given the information of the trauma. Visual acuity testing, and afferent pupillary defect are routinely performed. With the eyes with open wound, globe integrity might be compromised during examination; assessment should be limited to non-contact, non-invasive in nature. Even squeezing can jeopardize the eye, should be avoided. In traumatic eyes with perforating mechanism, lens removal is usually performed at the same time of treatment on the accompanied trauma on cornea or sclera, especially in cases that definite lens damage and severe inflammation in the anterior chamber due to the cortical material are suspected. However, it could be delayed after the primary closure of laceration on cornea or sclera until identification of the extent of damage of the lens or development of visually significant cataract.

In many occasions with open wound, visibility of the wound is poor due to hemorrhage in vitreous cavity and anterior chamber, primary closure alone could be the proper procedure at the time of

© Springer-Verlag Berlin Heidelberg 2016
W.S. Kim, K.H. Kim, *Challenges in Cataract Surgery*, DOI 10.1007/978-3-662-46092-4_8

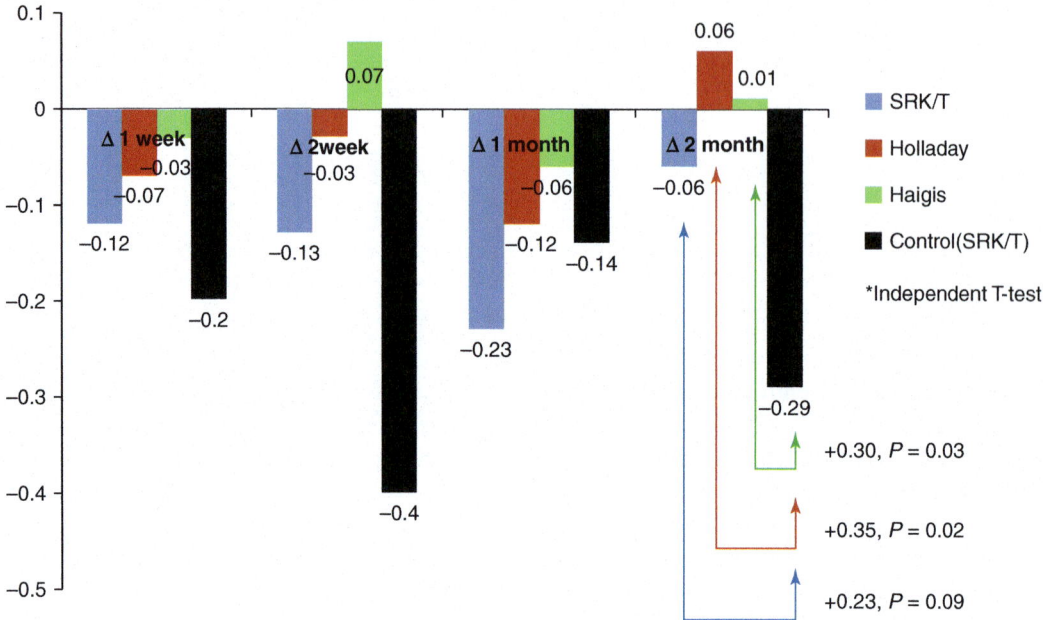

Fig. 8.1 Hyperopic shifting was found after phacoemulsification & in the bag IOL implantation in blunt traumatic cataract in our study. Compare to 1 week, average

+0.30 diopter of hyperopic change was found at postoperative 2 months in 34 eyes

primary surgery. CT scan can provide useful information when visibility of posterior segment is poor, such as suprachoroidal hemorrhage and detachment, presence and location of IOF.

For open wound, general anesthesia is standard approach in order not to disturb the orbital structure. Regional or topical anesthesia is chosen for closed wound in cooperative patient. Surgeon should discuss with the patient about the possible benefits and drawbacks of each anesthetic procedures before selection of anesthesia technique. For injuries with open globe and lacerated lens capsule, cataract extraction should be performed at the time of the open globe repair to remove all the liberated lens material from the eye to prevent postoperative lens induced uveitis and secondary glaucoma. Risk of ruptured anterior and posterior capsule is high, try not to remove too much of capsular leaflet, they should be spared to facilitate the secondary implantation of the IOL in the sulcus. Even the torn posterior capsule to the equator with ragged margin will fuse to anterior capsule and provide a safe place to implant IOL in the sulcus (Fig. 8.1).

Intraoperative Considerations

If open wound is found, it should be secured watertight, before making an incision for cataract surgery. As I described in Chap. 11, in cases with zonular dialysis or penetrating wound, incisions are made on the quadrant with attached zonules and capsules to put vitreous face in remote location from irrigating fluid.

Bottle height, irrigation flow rate, and vacuum are set at minimum ("slow phaco") to minimize the disturbance of orbital structure during phaco procedure. Retentive viscoelstics dispersive viscoelastics such as Viscoat®(Alcon, USA) are more helpful in tamponading vitreous face and protection of vitreous hydration, and protection of corneal endothelium. Dispersive agents are more difficult to remove at the completion of the surgery and postoperative IOP rise is frequent. Cohesive viscoelastics, Healon 5® or Healon GV® (Pharmacia, Sweden) are preferred by the author, because they are easier to remove at the completion of the surgery compared to dispersive

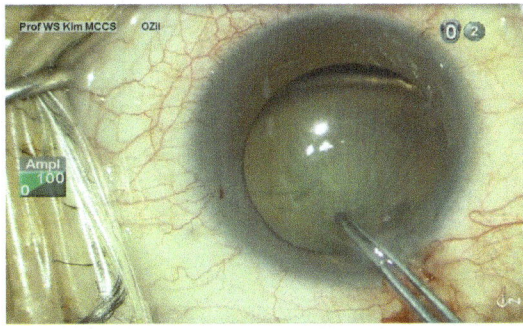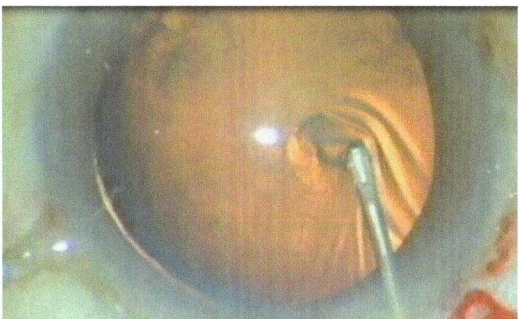

Fig. 8.2 Anterior capsular wrinkling during CCC

viscoelastics. When viscoelastic is used to between capsule and lens material I wound recommend to use Viscoat® or Healon® because they separate the capsule from lens material and keep the capsule back to its position. In order to tamponade the vitreous face, both of the viscoelastics are helpful, however, removal of Healon 5® is easier at the completion of the surgery. If all the parameters are set at low level, there is less disturbance of orbital content during phaco procedure, and surgery becomes more controllable. I prefer to use Healon GV® at low parameter setting, to make removal of viscoelastic easier, and to make immediate postoperative period more comfortable.

During capsulotomy, close observation is necessary to detect any big wrinkling on anterior capsular surface, which is a sign of loose zonule (Fig. 8.2). In cases with mature white cataract, use of capsule staining and space retaining viscoelastics is useful. I do not recommend to use capsule staining in cases with large zonular dialysis or in cases with large double penetration of lens capsule with visible vitreous face, because the dye will get access to the vitreous cavity through zonular defect or capsular defect, stain the vitreous fibers, and red reflex becomes diminished. Some surgeons prefer to "plug" the vitreous face with dispersive viscoelastics before applying capsular staining in these cases with open vitreous face. In our practice, Indocyanine green and trypan blue in use because of their safety profile and effectiveness. Staining technique is described in Chap. 1. Staining can easily delineate the ragged margin of anterior capsule due to penetrating trauma. Use of tangential illumination of

endoilluminator probe facilitate visualization of lens capsule with white cataract or any cases with poor red reflex [2].

Even though intact CCC margin has the highest mechanical strength, can opener capsulotomy or use of vitrector is used in occasions. I found it easier to use capsule staining and space retaining viscoelastic materials in creation of successful CCC in cases with mature cataract. As the age of the traumatic cataract is usually younger than that of senile cataract and progression of cataract is rapid, CCC techniques are much similar to that of pediatric cataract.

For the capsular tension ring to stay in the capsular bag, integrity of the capsule is important, if there is penetrating wound in posterior capsule, which did not or cannot be converted to CCC, try not to use capsular tension ring.

Postoperative Considerations

– Topical broad spectrum antibiotic : (levofloxacin 0.5 % [Cravit®, Santen, Japan] or moxifloxacin 0.5 % [Vigamox®, Alcon, USA] qid)

– Topical steroids : (prednisolone acetate 1 % [Pred forte®, Allergan, USA] qid, routinely)

– Topical NSAIDs : (bromfenac [Bronuck®, Taejoon pharm., Korea] bid or flurbiprofen sodium 0.03 % [Flurbiprofen®, Basch&Lomb, USA] qid)

- May require treatment of increased intra-ocular pressure: dorzolamide/timolol [Cosopt®, Santen, Japan] bid, brimonidine tartrate 0.1 % [Alphagan-P®, Allergan, USA] bid, Carbonic anhydrase inhibitor, acetazolamide [Acetazol®, Hanlim pharm., Korea]

References

1. Muga R, Maul E. The management of lens damage in perforating corneal lacerations. Br J Ophthalmol. 1978;62:784–7.
2. Steinert RF. Chapter 6 Cataract surgery. 3rd ed. Philadelphia: Saunders; 2010. p. 355.

Iris Surgeries

9

Iris abnormalities frequently occur as a result of penetrating trauma, blunt injuries, surgical injuries (most frequently after cataract surgeries) and as congenital reason such as in cases with iris coloboma, and corectopia.

Iris defects cause decreased functional vision and increased photic phenomenon. When IOL is placed in the defective iris, photic phenomenon and lens edge effect become increased, due to smaller size of IOL compared to human lens. When performing cataract surgeries in eyes with enlarged or defective pupil, the patients should be warned about the possibility of photic phenomenon and lens edge effect then additional need for iris surgeries during cataract surgery or afterwards.

Preoperative Considerations

Before placing a suture, careful inspection of torn iris and planning of reconstruction should be performed. Take cautions to preserve as much iris tissue as possible to use it as a building block for pupil reconstruction, unless iris tissue is infected. In many occasions, iris tends to protrude outside the eye through corneal laceration, minimal corneal suturing is needed before placing the iris back to the anterior chamber.

If adhesion of iris is found, it can be mobilized using a round spatula or viscoelastic agent (visco-dissection). Before placing a suture, shape of iris damage should be evaluated meticulously. If iris trauma occurred after surgical trauma (most frequently during phaco-surgery), posterior pigmented layer of iris are more easily aspirated through phaco tip, and frequently lost. Not infrequently torn iris segments are flipped over, should be repositioned before suturing. Posterior surface of the non-pigmented epithelium is more smooth and shinny. When radial tear and iridodialysis is present together, I prefer to correct radial tear first.

Radial Tearing with Ruptured Iris Sphincter Muscle (Figs. 9.1, 9.2, and 9.3)

For radial tear, first suture should close the pupil by putting torn sphincter muscle close together. Using long curved needle (Ethicon 10–0 Prolene polypropylene suture with CIF-4 needle), corneal punctures is made 3 clock hours apart from sphincter rupture. Then penetrate the closer lip of the sphincter muscle on sphincter rupture outside-in then the distal lip inside out. The needle tip is lead toward the other side of the cornea, then pull the needle outside of the eye leaving the needle thread. Needle is cut from the thread. 1-mm stab corneal incision is made on the quadrant of

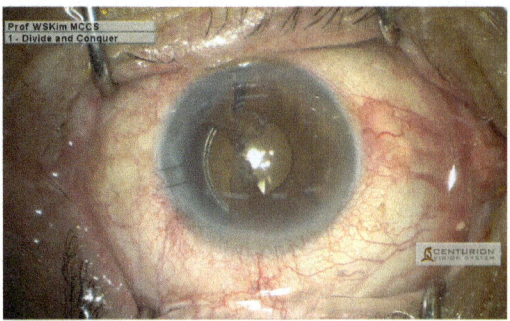

Fig. 9.1 After cataract surgery with IOL implantation, radial tear of iris and iridodialysis was found. The patient referred to clinic to repair iris damage. Part of iris fragment is turned upside down, pigment epithelium of iris is lost

pupillary sphincter rupture, mid-peripheral region. Reversely bent 30-Gauge needle is drawn inside the eye through the stab incision, and pull both sides of the thread outside the eye. Both ends are pulled and tied to secure a knot. 1-mm corneal incision usually does not need suturing, however, needs to be checked for water tightness. Corneal suturing should be considered if there's any possibility of leak is noticed.

Iridodialysis, Cyclodialysis (Figs. 9.4, 9.5, and 9.6)

In cases with iridodialysis, attachment of the detached iris is performed with long curved needle. Corneal stab incision is made 90° apart from planned suture site to have a secure access.(If the stab incision is too far, pressure is applied to the globe, and risk of lens damage is increased). Conjuntival incision is made on quadrant of dialysis. Pass the needle through corneal limbus on the quadrant of iris dialysis, through peripheral part of detached iris from behind. Draw the needle through a corneal stab incision on 90° apart. Needle is reintroduced into the anterior chamber,

pass the distal end of the detached iris1 ~ 1.5 clock apart antero-posteriorly, then pass the corneal limbus inside-out. Two ends of the suture are tied. Rotate the suture knot inside the eye to avoid knot exposure through conjunctiva.

When attach the iris to the sclera wall, I prefer to place it more anteriorly to compensate for shortened iris on the detached quadrant.

Detached iris tends to curl posteriorly, surgeon needs to catch the very end of the iris after ab-interno entry, to avoid serious shortening of the iris. If needle with two long-curved needles is used both ends of the needle can be passed through a paracentesis incision, through distal end of the iris 1–1.5 clock hour apart, though sclera wall, then both ends are tied on the sclera surface under conjunctiva.

Atonic Dilated Pupil/Pupillary Capturing (Figs. 9.7, 9.8, and 9.9)

Purse-String suture is used for atonic dialted pupil, and pupillary capturing of the iris. I prefer to place stab incisions on 12, 3, 6 and 9 o'clock position. Inject cohesive viscoelastics into anterior chamber. Introduce a long curved needle through the stab incision on 12 o'clock position, penetrate the stroma of iris on superotemporal quadrant, pull the needle out through stab incision in proximity.

Same procedure is repeated at each quadrant until the needle passes out through the stab incision on 12 o'clock position. Suture is pulled and tied to make pupil diameter of 3–4 mm.

Artificial Iris

Although not available in our current practice, many different kinds of artificial irises are used. If permanent defect that cannot be close using sutures, artificial Irises are used [1–3].

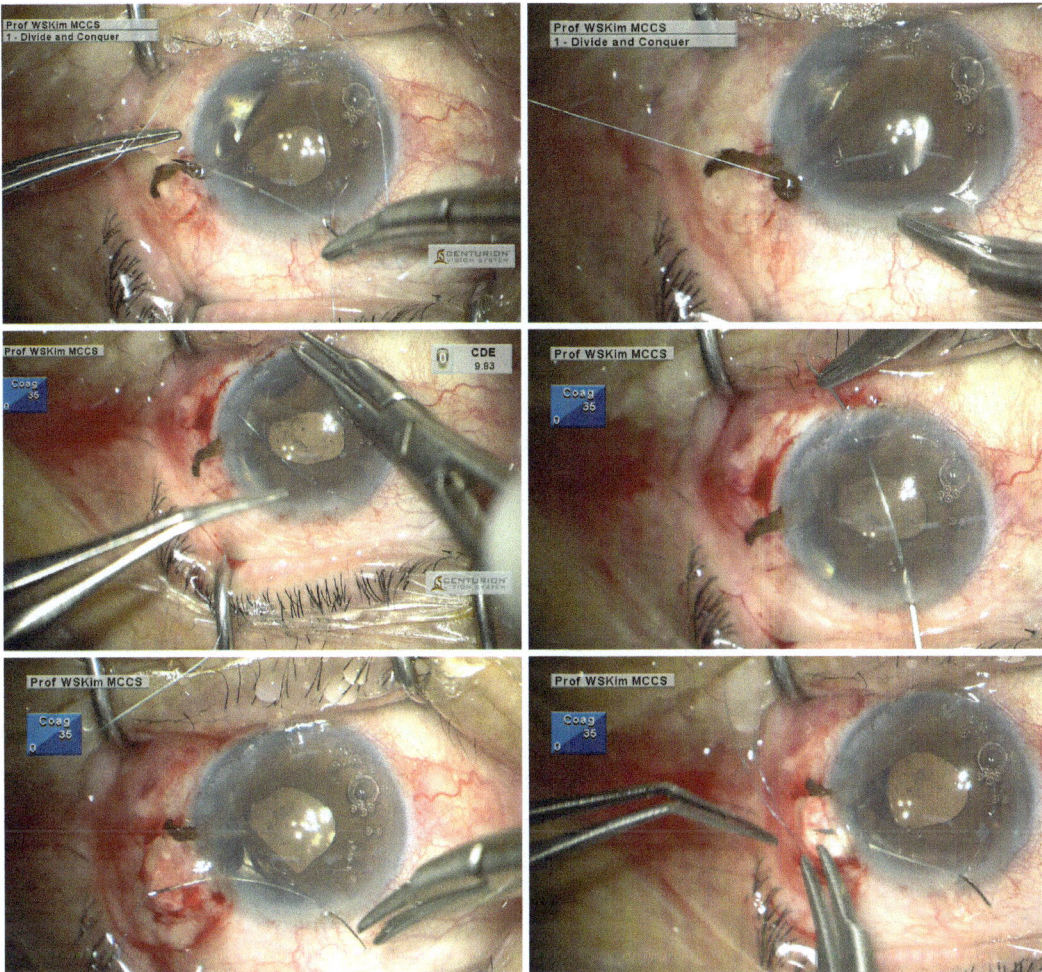

Fig. 9.2 (*Top Left*) Torn iris is prolapsed to corneal incision site. Long curved needle is inserted into anterior chamber to suture torn iris. (*Top Right*) Separated iris is tighed at 3 o clock, outside of anterior chamber (*Middle Left*) Sutured iris is inserted back into anterior chamber. 4 o clock detached iris root was suture toward cornea. (*Middle Right*) Inferior side detached iris root is anchored to cornea using long curved needle. (*Bottom Left*) Long curved needle is inserted at 2 o clock to anchor detached iris root. (*Bottom Right*) Long curved needle get out from anterior chamber through 12 o clock, and inserted again into anterior chamber to anchor iris root at 2 o clock

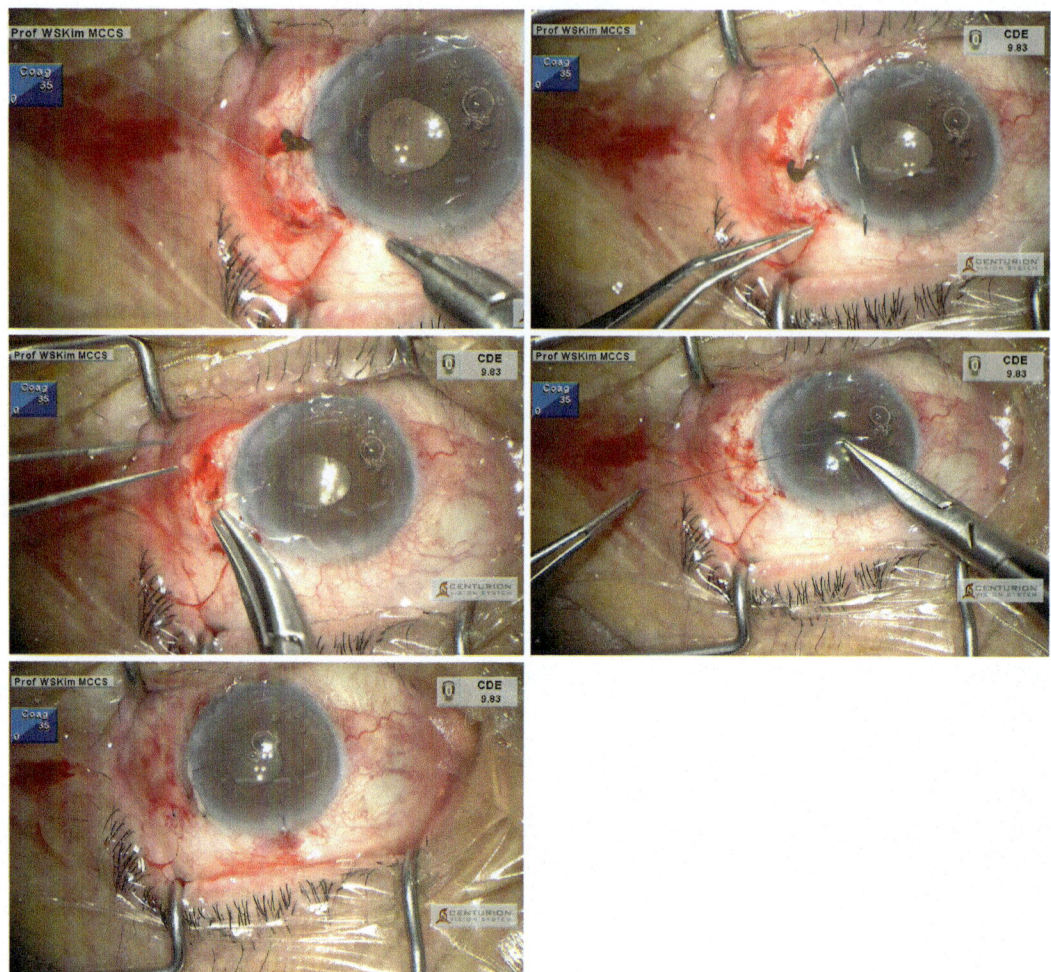

Fig. 9.3 (*Top left*) Suture is tightened at 2 o clock. (*Top right*) Long curved needle is inserted into anterior chamber to suture torn iris near papillary margin. (*Middle Left*) Temporal side cornea and iris root suture is made. (*Middle Right*) Cornea suture is made at 3 clock. (*Bottom*) After pupilloplasty, torn iris and iridodialysis is repaired

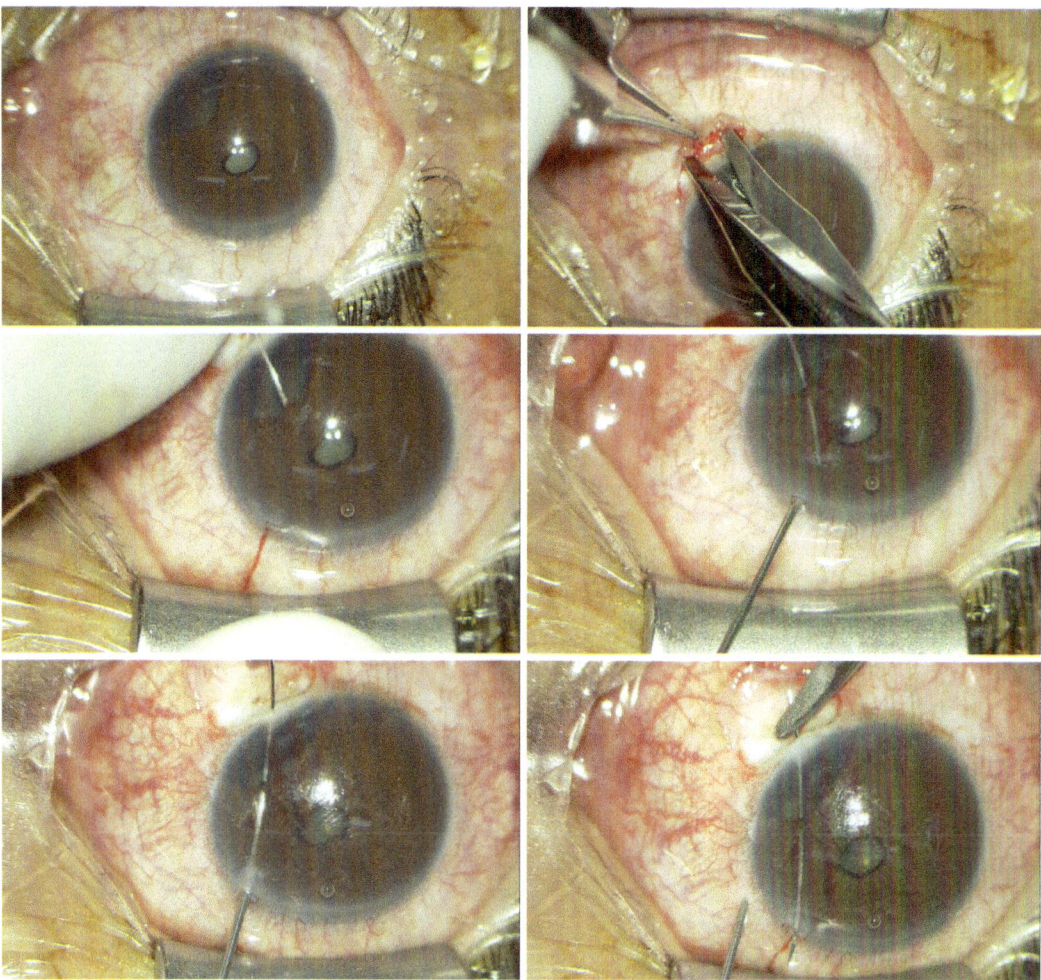

Fig. 9.4 (*Top Left*) Iridodialysis is found at 3~6 o clock position. (*Top Right*) Conjunctival peritomy is made on the quadrant of iridodialysis. (*Middle Left*) Long curved needle is inserted into anterior chamber. (*Middle Right*) With the long curved needle penetrated peripheral part of the dialyzed iris, 27G needle is inserted through paracen- tesis incision to dock the long curved needle. (*Bottom Left*) Two needle is docked in anterior chamber. (*Bottom Right*) Long curved needle is drawn out from the anterior chamber through paracentesis incision, where the docking needle was inserted

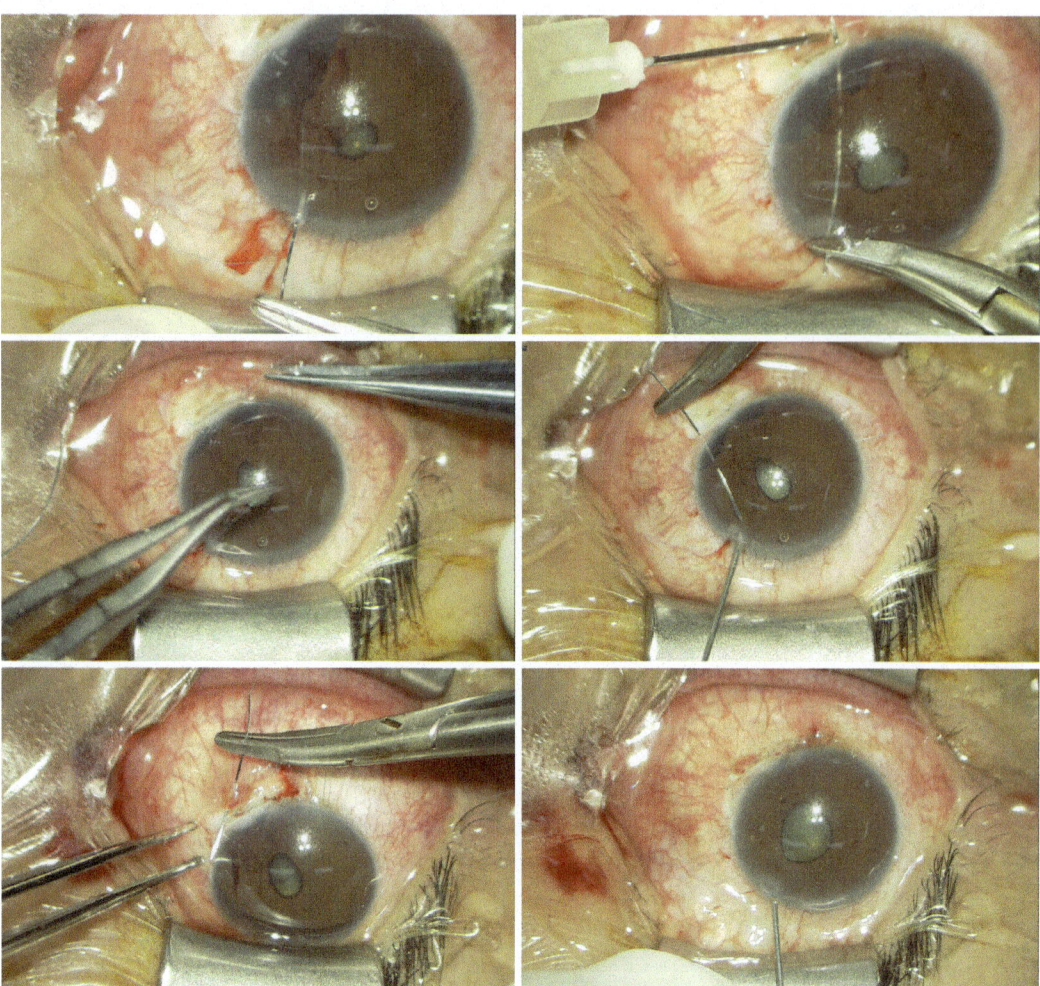

Fig. 9.5 (*Top Left*) Long curved needle is re-inserted into anterior chamber though the paracentesis. (*Top Right*) The long curved needle penetrate the peripheral part of the dialyzed iris antero-posteriorly 1 ~ 1.5 clock hours apart. The needle then penetrate the sclera from inside out. (*Middle Left*) Suture is tightened at 5 o clock position. (*Middle Right*) Same procedure is repeated on other quadrants of dialyzed iris. (*Bottom Left*) Conjunctival suture is performed. (*Bottom Right*) By replacing detached iris root toward cornea, iris dragging is minimized, creates cosmetically better result

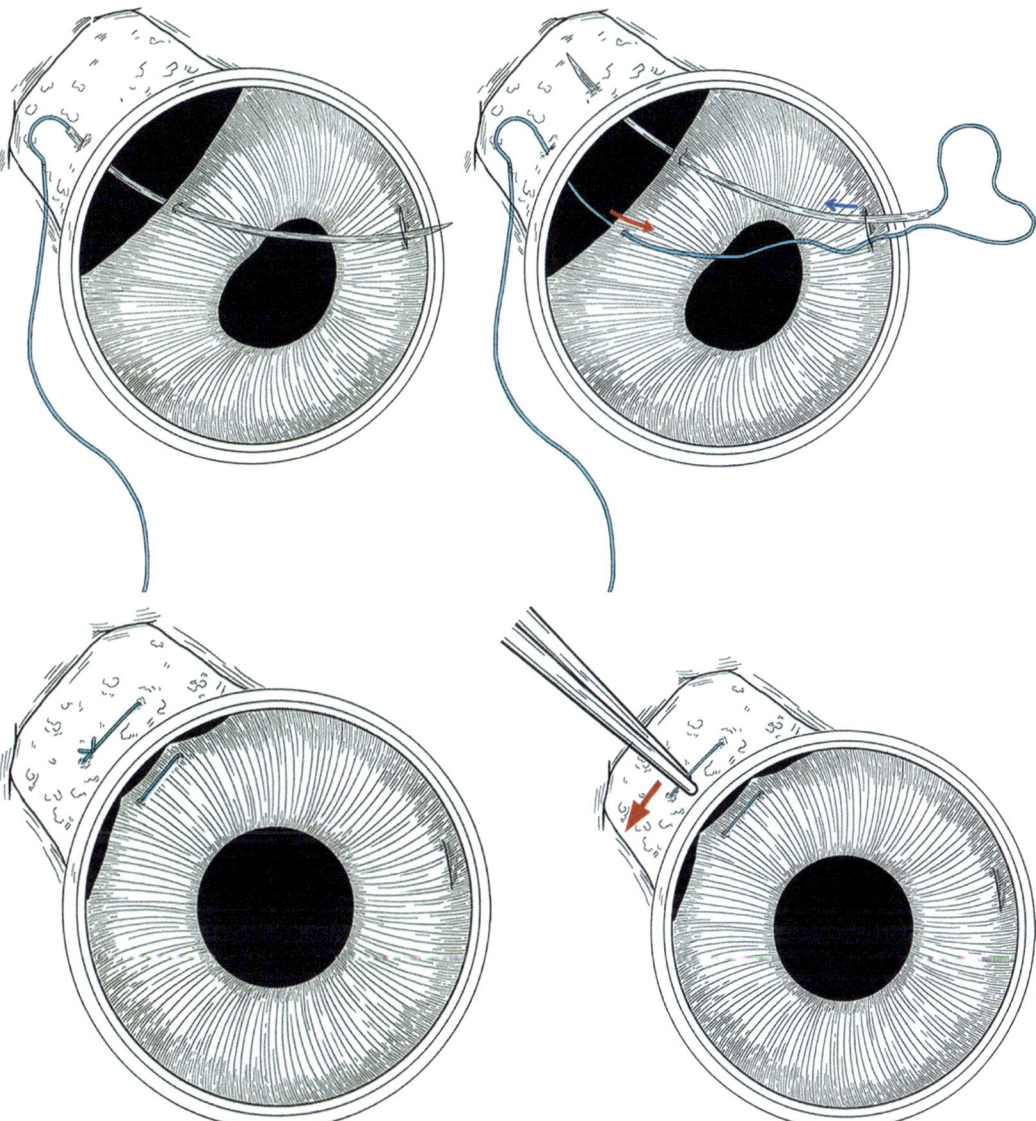

Fig. 9.6 Illustrations of iridodialysis repairing. (*Top Left*) The long curved needle penetrate the sclera, peripheral part of the dialyzed iris. (*Top Right*) Then the needle re- entered to anterior chamber, using corneal incision site and penetrate the sclera from inside out to anchor iris root toward cornea. (*Bottom*) The suture is buried

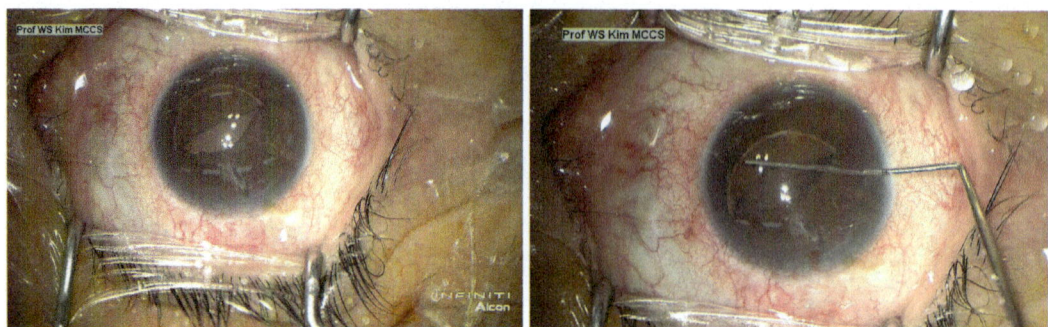

Fig. 9.7 (*Left*) IOL Optic capture is found at inferior side. (*Right*) Captured IOL is replaced using instrument. (Sinsky hook)

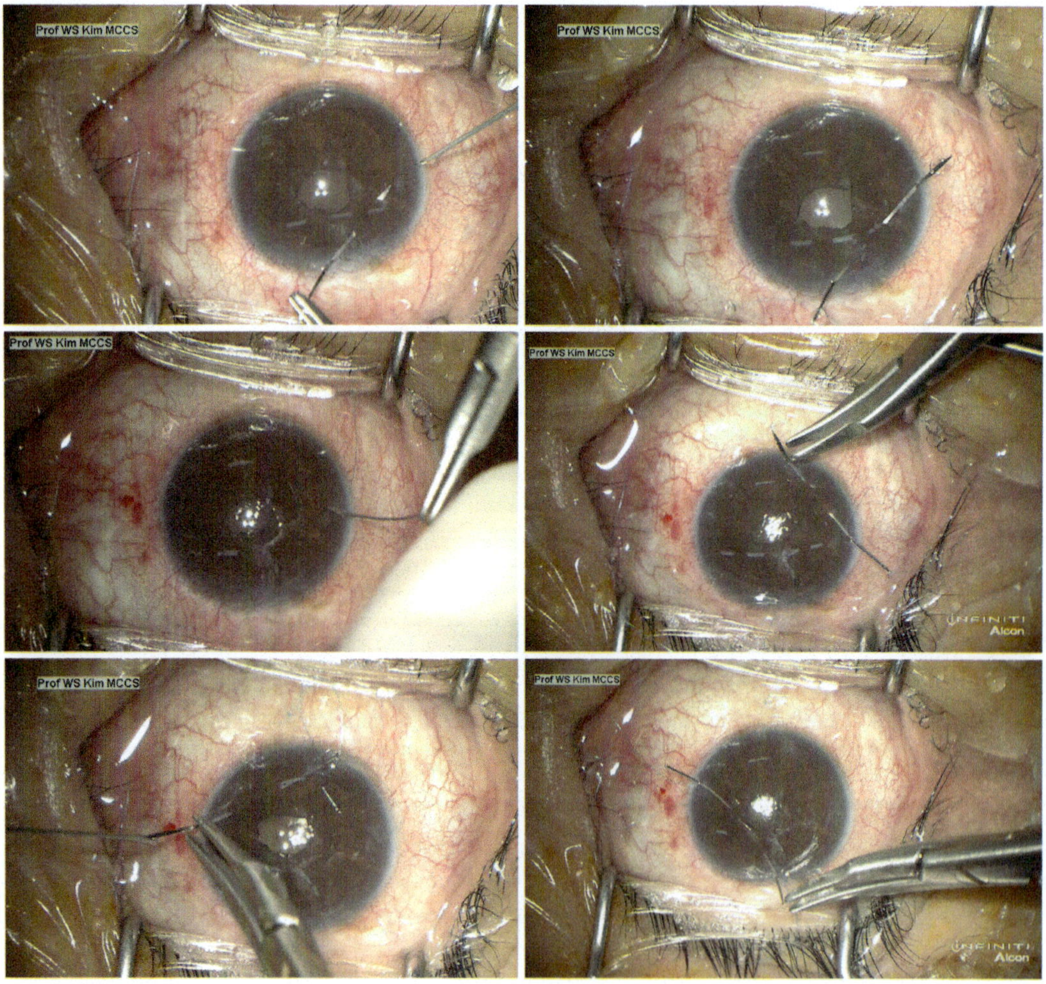

Fig. 9.8 Iris purse string suture is done at four quadrant

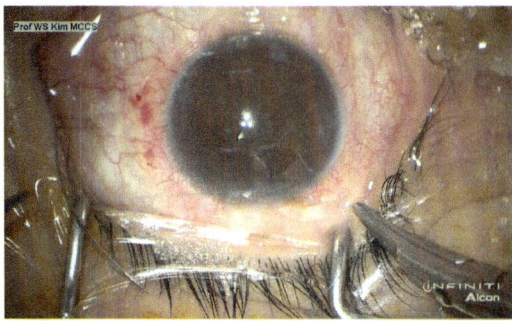

Fig. 9.9 After purse string suture, suture is tightened at superior side

References

1. Mayer CS, Hoffmann AE. Surgical treatment with an artificial iris. Ophthalmology. 2015;112:865–8.
2. Burk SE, Da Mata AP, Snyder ME, et al. Prosthetic iris implantation for congenital, traumatic, or functional iris deficiencies. J Cataract Refract Surg. 2001;27:1732–40.
3. Mavrikakis I, Mavrikakis E, Syam PP, et al. Surgical management of iris defects with prosthetic iris devices. Eye (Lond). 2005;19:205–9.

Dislocation of Crystalline Lens and Marfan's Syndrome

10

Lens dislocation is caused by trauma, hereditary, or spontaneous. If the patient has serious blunt injury to the operating eye, we have to be prepared for lens dislocation during surgery even if we cannot find any defect of zonules or displacement of crystalline lens.

Trauma is the most frequent cause (more than 50%) of crystalline lens dislocation. Heritable lens dislocation includes Marfan syndrome, homocystinuria, Weil-Marchesani syndrome and many other genetic conditions. Conditions that stretches and weakens the zonules such as hypermature cataract, angle closure glaucoma with very shallow chamber are also common causes of crystalline lens dislocation.

Marfan syndrome has triad symptoms of ectopia lentis, cardiovascular abnormalities, and skeletal abnormalities. Ectopia lentis is the most frequent symptom (70–80%) and always bilateral, and lens shifting is upward and temporally (Fig. 10.1) [1, 2]. It is autosomal dominantly inherited and expression is variable. Because of their AD inherence, it is required to inform the family about strong genetic penetrance.

Preoperative Considerations

Preoperatively, phacodonesis, iridodonesis, visible lens equater, scalloping of the lens capsule, herniated vitreous, visible defect of zonules can be found. Phacodonesis is readily noticed before dilation of pupil because dilation stabilize the ciliary body and iris. If the lens is inferiorly displaced with the effect of gravity, it is a sign of extreme zonular weakness (360 degrees) or defect. In Marfan syndrome, zonules are not defective but elongated and weakened therefore thickness of the lens is increased on the quadrant of the elongated zonule.

Careful history taking is important, they usually underestimate the impact or even the presence of previous ocular injuries. If there's any history of ocular trauma, the patient should be examined in supine position or tilt the head backwards in sitting position using hand slitlamp. Gravity pulls lens downwards and defect is usually notable.

In planning the surgery it is critical to detect the quadrant of zonular dialysis. Under slitlamp examination, quadrant with widest gap between iris and the anterior lens capsule is the quadrant with defective zonule. Pressing the circumference of the limbus using cotton tip applicator can detect the areas of zonular defect. If the lens does not move in accordance with the depressed limbus, there's the defect. During corneal incision, as the anterior chamber fluid egresses and lens movement is excessive. During capsulorhexis, we find big wrinkles on the quadrant of the zonule weakness, because the zonules cannot readily counteract the pulling force created by capsulorhesis forceps.

© Springer-Verlag Berlin Heidelberg 2016
W.S. Kim, K.H. Kim, *Challenges in Cataract Surgery*, DOI 10.1007/978-3-662-46092-4_10

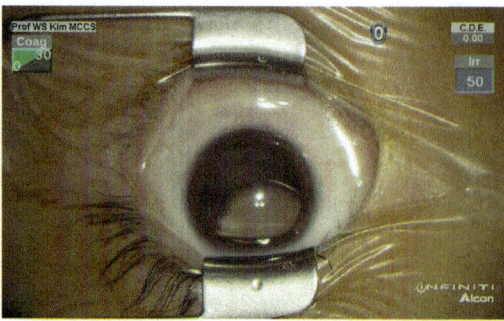

Fig. 10.1 This Marfan syndrome patient has ectopia lentis and the lens shifting is upward and temporally

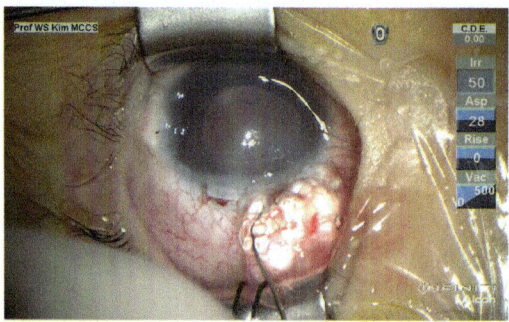

Fig. 10.2 In the case of cohesive viscoelastics, they can be removed easily by injecting BSS into anterior chamber through incision

OVD

If vitreous face is exposed, dispersive viscoelastics are preferred by many surgeons, because they tamponade the vitreous and keep it back. However, dispersive viscoelastics placed on the vireous face is difficult to remove at the completion of the surgery and cause IOP elevation after surgery not infrequently. If cohesive viscoelastics are used, they can be removed easily by injecting BSS into anterior chamber through incision (Fig. 10.2). Soft shell technique is preferred by many surgeons to have the benefits of using two different kinds of viscoelastics [3].

Intraoperative Considerations

Progressive Severe Zonulopathy: Marfan Syndrome

Marfan syndrome is the most frequent congenital cause of ectopia lentis, which occurs in

80–90 % of affected individuals. Zonular dialysis is known to be progressive and profound in this condition. In patients with mild to moderate lens subluxation, a CTR can be employed. However, posterior capsular opacification (PCO) and late IOL dislocation secondary to progressive fibrous adhesions between the zonular and capsular complexes can occur at a later date [4, 5].

To manage severe lens subluxation, an IOL can be sutured to the scleral wall after intracapsular cataract extraction or pars plana lensectomy. However, postoperative vitreoretinal complications and severe astigmatism are known complications after such surgery. Therefore, we proposed a novel surgical technique in which the lens is removed through a small incision, without breaking the anterior vitreous face, and an IOL is sutured to the sclera.

In this technique, after formation of two fornix-based conjunctival incisions at the 6- and 12-o'clock positions, half-thickness triangular scleral flaps are constructed 180° apart. A stab incision and a limbal incision of 2.8 mm are made in the quadrant where the zonules are intact. Using a bent needle, a puncture is made on the surface of the anterior capsule in the quadrant of the intact zonules. The capsulorrhexis is completed using capsulorrhexis forceps. I try to make large capsulorhexis to prevent capsule contraction. When zonule's traction force is decreased, control of directing CCC becomes less challenging. Advantages of large CCC are prevention of capsular contraction that is fairly common with weak zonule, less zonular tension during lens nucleus manipulation, and tighter sealing when pulled with iris retractors.

Iris rector pulling the CCC margin and iris together can seal the gap between the iris and lens, then can stabilize the anterior chamber. Iris retractors are inserted though stab incisions located closer to the iris attachment rather than clear cornea in order not to exert too much traction on the capsulorhexis margin and iris. 5 or 6 iris retractors can be inserted to distribute the tension exterted on each retractor and capsule to minimize the risk of capsular tear and also to prevent inflow of the BSS through the gap to the vitreous cavity. Therefore, the surgery can be performed in a stable, nicely distended capsular bag rather than continuously fluctuating anterior chamber with wrinkling capsular bags that keeps coming closer to the phaco tip.

Another advantage of using iris retractor is creation of complete compartmentalization. Complete compartmentalization can prevent or minimize vitreous hydration and vitreous herniation, however, if vitreous is present at any stage of the operation, it should be removed using "dry" vitrectomy using automatic vitrector and viscoelastics. For this purpose I prefer to use minimal amount of cohesive viscoelasitcs which can be easily removed at the completion of the surgery using irrigation rather than using I&A device.

Complete hydrodissection and hydrodelineation are then performed to minimize potential zonular damage during manipulation of the lens. Phacoemulsification and/or aspiration are performed with low bottle height and low vacuum settings.

After complete removal of the lens material, a cohesive OVD is injected through the loose zonules behind the capsular bag to separate the posterior capsule from the anterior vitreous face (Fig. 10.3a). A bent needle is used to create a puncture in the posterior capsule; intraocular scissors and capsulorrhexis forceps are then employed to remove the central part of the capsule.

In the process of pushing the vitreous face using OVD, the remaining elongated zonules and capsular remnants indicate the level of the vitreous face. A PC-7 needle (Alcon) is passed through the limbal incision, across the chamber, and above the vitreous face toward the ciliary sulcus at the 6-o'clock position under the scleral flap (Fig. 10.3b). The location of the needle can be detected by elevation of the sclera as the needle tip is gently pushed toward the outside (Fig. 10.4).

The needle is next passed to the exterior. The haptic of the IOL is sutured to the other end of the needle and then inserted into the anterior chamber. The trailing haptic is sutured to the other end of a PC-7 needle, and the needle sutures under the flap at the 12-o'clock position.

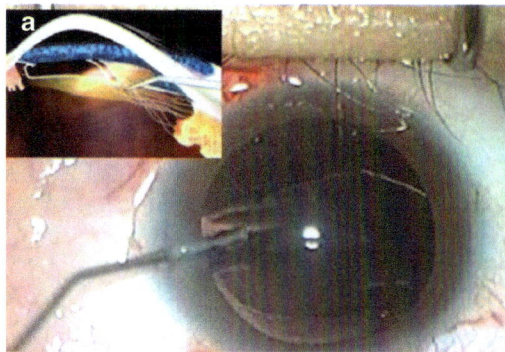

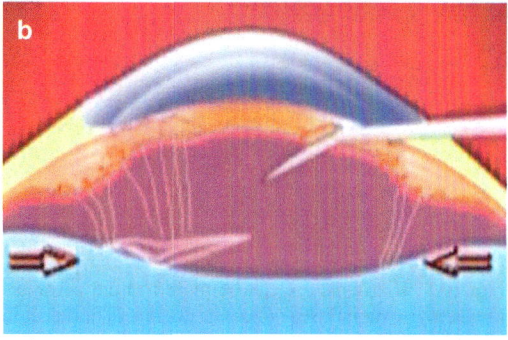

Fig. 10.3 Transscleral IOL fixation with preservation of the anterior vitreous in the treatment of ectopia lentis in a patient with Marfan syndrome. An OVD is injected through the loose zonules to separate the posterior capsule from the anterior vitreous face (**a**). Because residual zonules and capsular remnants indicate the level of the anterior vitreous face (*arrows*), a needle can be passed across the anterior chamber to the ciliary sulcus on the opposite side without breaking the anterior vitreous face (**b**)

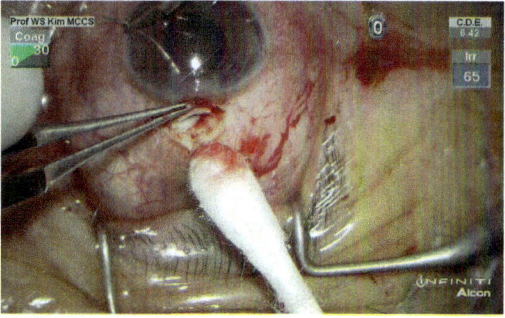

Fig. 10.4 The location of the needle can be detected by elevation of the sclera as the needle tip is gently pushed toward the outside

Scleral and limbal incisions are secured with 10–0 nylon sutures, and scleral flaps and conjunctival incisions are closed with 10–0 nylon sutures.

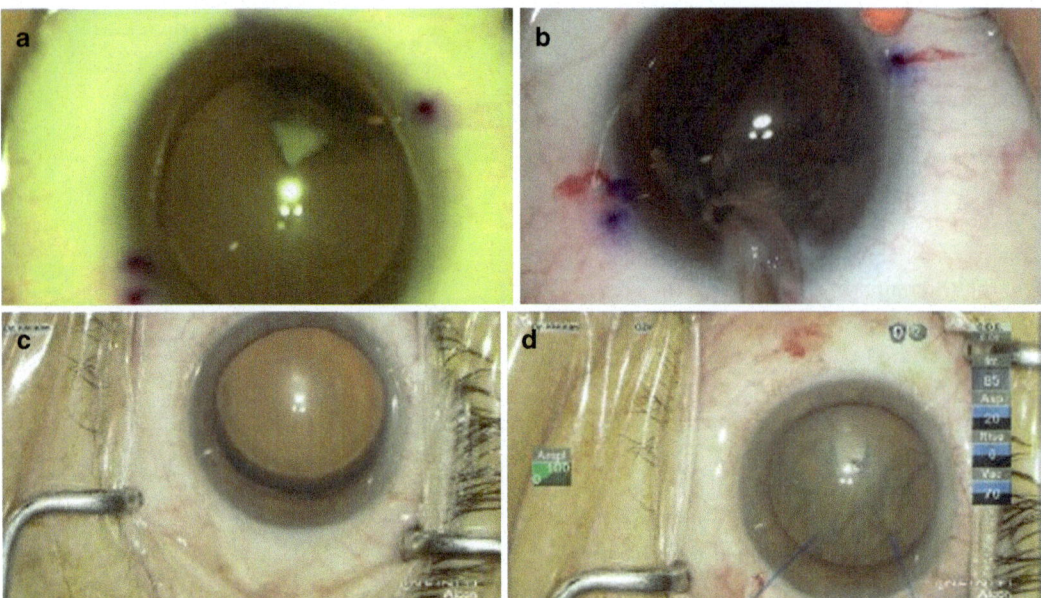

Fig. 10.5 Iris retractors can be placed at the capsulorrhexis edge over the area of zonular weakness or defect to stabilize a loose capsular-zonular complex during surgery. Case examples: A zonular defect associated with lens coloboma was detected (**a**), and iris retractors were used to bridge the gap effectively and prevent vitreous prolapse through the zonular defect during surgery (**b**). Profound zonular dialysis and lens dislocation after blunt trauma was observed (**c**), and iris retractors could have been used to stabilize the capsularlens complex during the entire operation (**d**)

Nonprogressive Zonulopathy: Congenital Lens Coloboma and Traumatic Crystalline Lens Dislocation

Zonulopathy in eyes with congenital lens coloboma and traumatic crystalline lens dislocation is known to be nonprogressive, although the amount of zonular defect or weakness varies according to disease entity and severity. These patients may be good candidates for the use of iris retractors instead of endocapsular devices.

Iris retractors can be placed at the capsulorrhexis edge over the area of zonular weakness or defect to stabilize the loose capsular-zonular complex during surgery (Fig. 10.5). However, close attention should be paid to the risk of inadvertent dislodging of the iris retractor and resultant anterior capsular tear. To reduce these risks when working with iris retractors, an adequately sized capsulorrhexis is of utmost importance. If the capsulorrhexis margin is small, the hook may drag on the capsulorrhexis edge and result in a capsular tear or dislodging of the hook.

Another strategy to minimize the risk of capsular tears is to use the iris retractor to hook the anterior capsule and the iris together. The iris stroma can be the buttress for the tension on the capsule by the tip of the retractor and, consequently, lessen the risk of capsular tears or dislodging of the retractor. An important factor in maintaining a stable position of the retractor is the location of the paracentesis used for its insertion. A paracentesis made near the limbus may be more advantageous for the iris retractor to be parallel to the iris plane and therefore maximize the stability of the retractor compared with one made far from the limbus (Fig. 10.6).

After the lens is removed using retractors, a loose capsular-zonular complex can be stabilized by in-the-bag implantation of an IOL with rigid

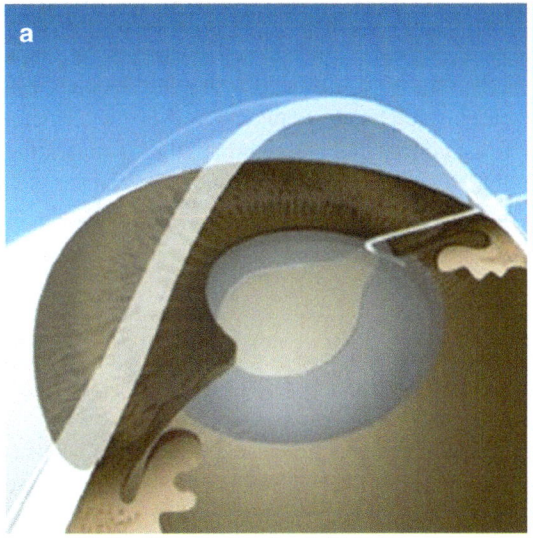

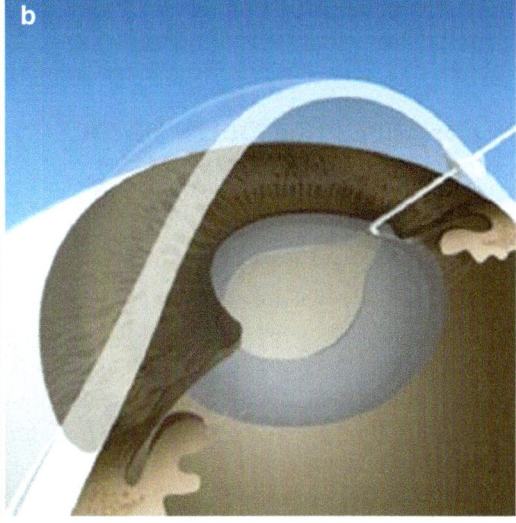

Fig. 10.6 Possible positions of an iris retractor according to insertion site are shown. A paracentesis made near the limbus may be more advantageous for the iris retractor to be parallel to the iris plane (**a**), thereby maximizing the stability of the retractor, compared with one made far from the limbus (**b**)

haptics, such as three-piece IOLs with acrylic or silicone optics and PMMA haptics. In eyes with a localized zonular defect, we prefer that the IOL haptics be oriented toward the zonular dialysis. The haptics can thus expand the capsular equator and buttress the weak area in a similar way to an endocapsular device. For larger defects, by contrast, orientation of the haptics toward intact zonules is more advantageous because this can help maintain healthy zonules in the event of late capsular contracture (Video).

Risk of Late IOL Dislocation

Despite these steps, larger zonular defects still carry the risk of late in-the-bag dislocation. However, IOL dislocation can be treated by repositioning the dislocated lens using scleral or iris fixation.

Although IOL fixation to the iris has the advantage of requiring a shorter operation time, it also has several drawbacks, including increased rates of induced astigmatism, less stable refraction, and immediate and recurring postoperative inflammation [4]. Therefore, scleral fixation is

our preference in the event of in-the-bag IOL dislocation.

Additionally, we incorporate primary posterior continuous curvilinear capsulorrhexis creation during the operation in eyes with zonular dialysis in an attempt to minimize the risk of late capsular instability. The use of a posterior continuous curvilinear capsulorrhexis in cataract surgery can improve postoperative refractive stability by reducing IOL displacement during postoperative capsular bag fibrosis and shrinkage [5].

Incision should be made away from the zonular dialysis, even the side port incisions better be placed on the attached quadrant, to minimize the chance to disturb the vitreous face.

Hydrodissection and hydrodelineation should be carefully performed in order not to exert additional injury, however, should be a complete hydrodissection to ensure efficient maneuverability of the lens nucleus.

Phaco setting should be low bottle height, low flow rate, and low vacuum. With high bottle height cause higher inflow rate into the eye and water can easily get access through the defective zonule and to the vitreous cavity. Hydrated vitreous can fluctuate or shallow the anterior chamber.

Implantation of the IOL (PMMA IOL, Foldable Acrylic IOL with PMMA Haptic)

Large CCC is needed because the weak or lost zonules cannot counteract contracting lens capsular bag initiated by the centripetal force of the contacting capsulorhexis margin. With contracting lens capsular bag, tension exerted on the zonule increases, and eventually detaches. IOLs with PMMA haptic is required to support the capsular bag against the contracting capsular bag.

Orientation of the IOL is also critical. With large CCC and one to two quadrant of zonular dialysis, IOLs are implanted with the tension line (longitudinal axis of the IOL) to meet the center of dialysis. 180 degrees zonular dialysis on inferior quadrant stays well than that on superior quadrant.

Even with 180 degrees zonular dialysis, IOL-capsular bag complex function like a plate after capsular fusion, Therefore, we can assess the stability of the IOL after 3–4 weeks of observation.

In cases with Marfan's syndrome, dislocated capsular bag was sutured using Cionni Ring CTR (capsular tension ring), however, capsular bag dislocation occurs during the course of the time due to progressive fibrotic changes pulling capsular bag upward and. Suture fixation using 9–0 or 8–0 Prolene of Cionni Ring was tried, but it will not keep the capsular bag for long, and globe distortion will create unwanted astigmatism.

In cases with blunt trauma, zonules on temporal and nasal sides are preferably broken due to direct and contra-coup injury. Not infrequently, zonule segments only on 12 and 6 o'clock positions are remained. Even with minimal zonular attachment cataract surgery can be performed using iris retractor and meticulous surgical procedures. After surgery, lens stability is increased by iridocapsular adhesions.

I prefer to use Acrylic IOL with PMMA haptic. Larger optic IOL which is more forgiving to small amount of decentration is preferred. Large

PMMA IOL which requires large incision increase risk of vitreous incarceration. Foldable soft IOLs with soft haptics should not be used in cases with weak zonule, because, they cannot resist contracting capsular bag, thus jeopardizing IOLs' stability. At the completion of the surgery, pupils should be constricted (using Miochol or Miostat) to search for any vitreous incarcerations.

CTR Capsular Tension Rings

Since the introduction of the original endocapsular device in 1991, there has been a progressive evolution of designs to help surgeons manage profound zonular weakness. Standard capsular tension rings (CTRs) may be useful in eyes with mild zonular instability such as small, localized zonular dialysis or mild diffuse zonular weakness. However, a standard CTR may not supply sufficient support to maintain the capsular bag in situations of profound or progressive zonular insufficiency, such as advanced pseudoexfoliation syndrome or Marfan syndrome. Further, in the setting of an anterior or posterior capsular tear, the risks of tear extension or loss of the device into the posterior segment limit the use of a standard CTR [1, 2].

With the advent of sclerally fixated devices such as modified CTRs and capsular tension segments (CTSs), adequate intraoperative or postoperative support can be achieved in eyes with profound zonular weakness. Additionally, these suturable endocapsular devices may be of optimal value in eyes with progressive zonulopathy, as they can be secured to the sclera. Further support can be achieved by combining devices.

A CTS can be implanted without a dialing technique; therefore, these devices may be useful in eyes with an incomplete rhexis, anterior capsular tear, or posterior capsular tear. As it provides support in the transverse plane when sutured to the sclera, a CTS may be used temporarily to provide intraoperative support of the capsule in an area of zonular weakness. In this situation, it can be hung from an inverted iris retractor placed through the eyelet of the CTS [1, 2].

Despite the advantages and utility of modified CTRs and CTSs, in Korea we have limited access to these devices due to the use of a diagnosis related group/prospective payment system and to lack of approvals by our country's regulatory body. Therefore, we have devised and performed alternative methods of stabilizing the capsule and IOL in eyes with large zonular dialysis of more than 4 clock hours and progressive zonulysis.

Postoperative Considerations

Even with large zonular dialysis, IOLs can be stabilized by irido-capsular adhesions. Eyes with atonic pupils cannot avoid irido-capsular synichiae.

Serious postoperative inflammations and CME can occur not infrequently and should be treated with topical corticosteroids.

Postoperative Medication

- Topical broad spectrum antibiotic: (Levofloxacin 0.5% [Cravit®, Santen, Japan] or Moxifloxacin 0.5% [Vigamox®, Alcon, USA] qid or Tobramycin 0.3% [Tobrex®, Alcon, USA] qid)
- Topical steroids: (Prednisolone acetate 1% [Pred forte®, Allergan, USA] q 1 h then tapered down to 4–8 weeks)
- Topical cycloplegics: (Tropicamide [Mydrin-P®, Santen, Japan] q 10 mins 6 times and atropine sulfate 1% [Isopto atropine®, Alcon, USA] qid for

2–4 weeks to continuously move the pupil then prevent synechiae formation).
- Topical NSAIDs: (Bromfenac [Bronuck®, Taejoon pharm., Korea] bid or Flurbiprofen sodium 0.03% [Flurbiprofen®, Basch&Lomb, USA] qid)
- May require treatment of increased intraocular pressure: Dorzolamide/timolol [Cosopt®, Santen, Japan] bid, Brimonidine tartrate 0.1% [Alphagan-P®, Allergan, USA] bid, Carbonic anhydrase inhibitor, acetazolamide [Acetazol®, Hanlim pharm., Korea]

References

1. Koenig SB, Mieler WF. Management of ectopia lentis in a family with Marfan syndrome. Arch Ophthalmol. 1996;114:1058–61.
2. Zadeh N, Bernstein JA, Niemi AK, Dugan S, Kwan A, Liang D, Hyland JC, Hoyme HE, Hudgins L, Manning MA. Ectopia lentis as the presenting and primary feature in Marfan syndrome. Am J Med Genet A. 2011;155:2661–8.
3. Arshinoff SA. Dispersive-cohesive viscoelastic soft shell technique. J Cataract Refract Surg. 1999;25:167–73.
4. Vadalà P, Capozzi P, Fortunato M, DeVirgiliis E, Vadalà F. Intraocular lens implantation in Marfan's syndrome. J Pediatr Ophthalmol Strabismus. 2000;37:206–8.
5. Rodrigo BJ, Paulina LL, Francesc Mde R, Eduardo TT, Alejandro N. Intraocular lens subluxation in marfan syndrome. Open Ophthalmol J. 2014;8:48–50.

Intraocular Lens Dislocation, Intraocular Lens Exchange and Secondary Intraocular Lens Fixation

11

The incidence of intraocular lens (IOL) dislocation is increasing as with the changes in surgeons' preference to newer IOL designs, introduction of soft IOLs and increased number of pseudophakic population in these years. Late decenteration is more frequently found in cases with uveitis cataract, pseudoexfoliation syndrome, and previous vitrectomy. Since capsule fibrosis and shrinkage is more prominent when silicon IOL material is used than other PMMA or acrylic material, I tried to find the difference in incidence of late IOL dislocation between IOLs made of different materials. Although we could not find the diffierence in the incidence between the eyes with different material, I believe it safer not to use IOLs inducing serious capsule contraction when weak zonules are noticed.

Removal of IOL

If IOLs integrity is broken and cannot be used for iris or scleral fixation, IOL should be removed.

Using IOL cutter, IOL can be devided into halves. Cautions should be used not to cut the scleral side of the corneal incision while advancing the knife cutter. Protecting the corneal incision with spatula can be helpful.

It is wise to cut the IOL longitudinally to decrease damage to corneal endothelium. If IOL is cut partially in half and try to remove by rotating the IOL after tucking half of the IOL, other half inside the eye can push the iris root, bleeding

can occur. To avoid this complication, IOLs can be cut in many long pieces completely in the eye. Or quadrant of the IOL optic is removed first second quadrant of the optic is tucked into the corneal incision, then is rotated to remove the rest of IOL (Figs. 11.1a, b).

We prefer to break the bulky plate haptic IOLs by cutting them into multiple longitudinal pieces, while non-bulky IOLs can be broken otherwise.

For IOLs dislocated in mid-vitreous or on retina, pars plana vitrectomy should be considered. IOLs are brought to anterior chamber during vitrectomy procedure.

IOL Dislocation and Scleral Fixation of IOL

There are several three-piece and one-piece IOLs designed for placement in the ciliary sulcus as well as in the capsular bag when anterior or posterior capsular support is insufficient. These IOLs have enough length and angulation, can be fixed to the sclera with various surgical techniques.

Preoperative Considerations

Preoperatively patients are examined at supine position, to evaluate the site of the attachment of the IOL. Knowing the location of the attachment of the IOL, and the type of subluxated or dislocated IOL is important in planning the relocation

© Springer-Verlag Berlin Heidelberg 2016
W.S. Kim, K.H. Kim, *Challenges in Cataract Surgery*, DOI 10.1007/978-3-662-46092-4_11

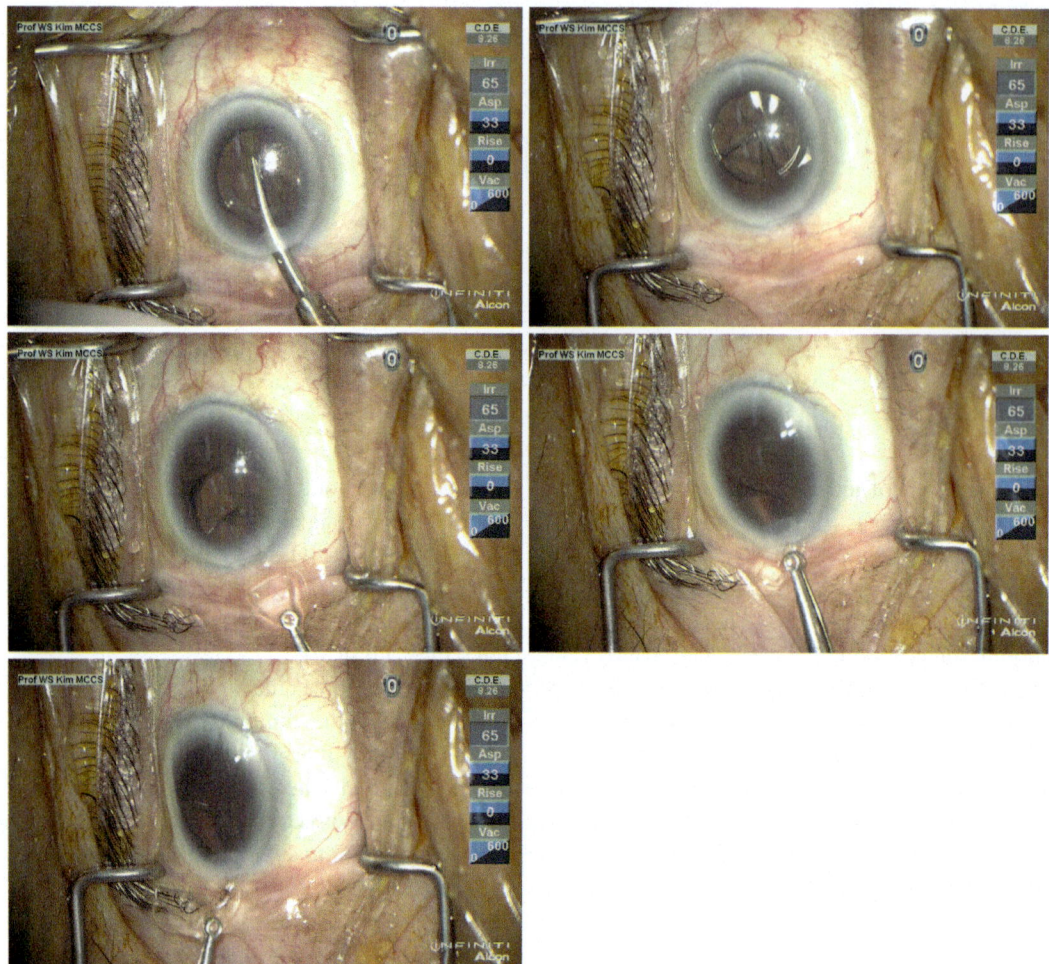

Fig. 11.1 IOLs can be cut in many long pieces completely in the eye. Or quadrant of the IOL optic is removed first second quadrant of the optic is tucked into the corneal incision, then is rotated to remove the rest of IOL

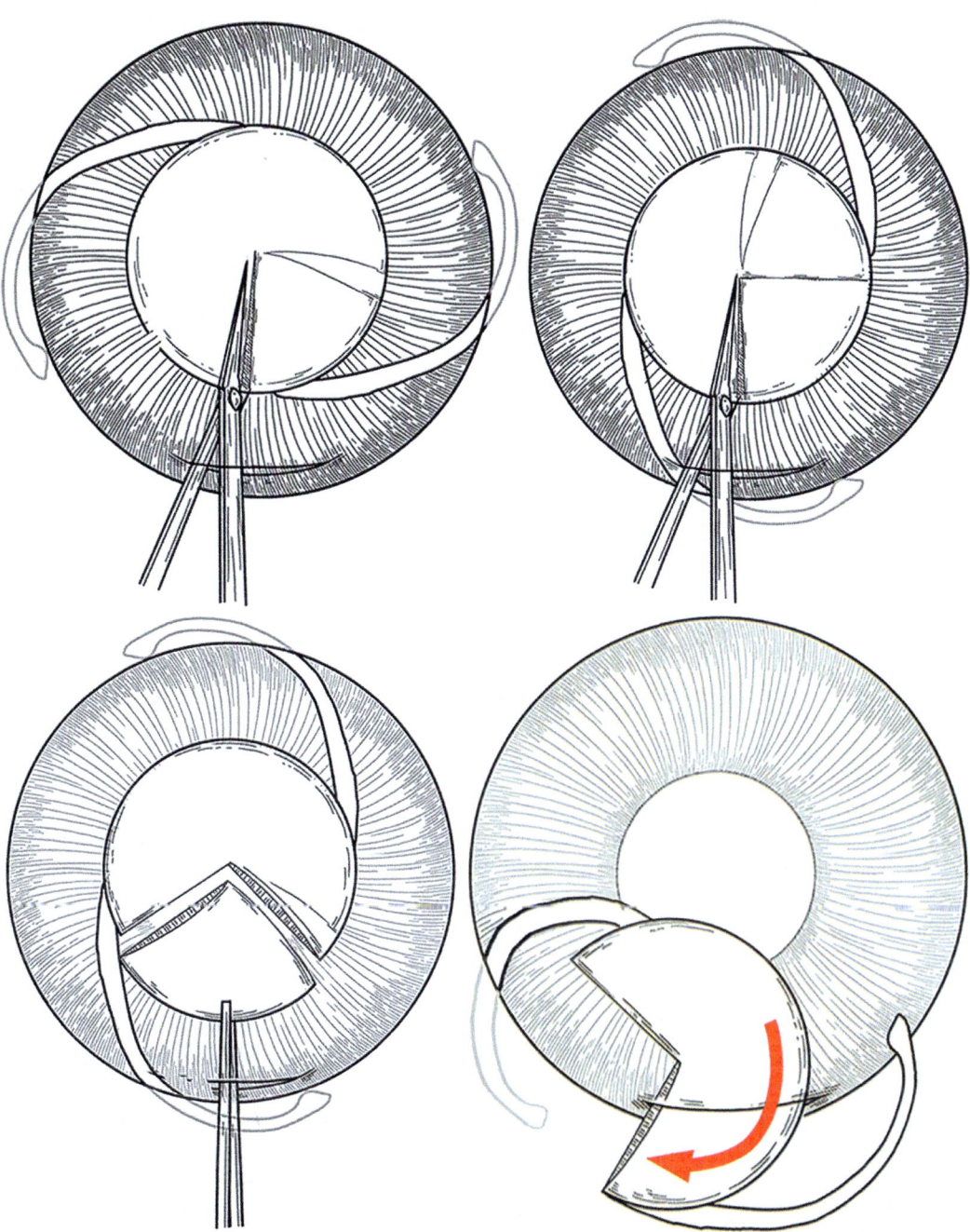

Fig. 11.1 (continued)

of the IOL. If there is firm attachment on one side (usually on the longest axis of the IOL-capsule complex), one point fixation of the IOL is my preference. Attachment of the IOL is checked by pressing the globe inward at the level of ciliary sulcus 360 degrees with cotton tip applicator.

Synchronous IOL movement can be found when we press the globe on the attached location, while we cannot find IOL movement when we press the globe on the detached quadrant (Fig. 11.2). For the IOL suitable for scleral fixation (PMMA or foldable IOL with PMMA haptic with overall

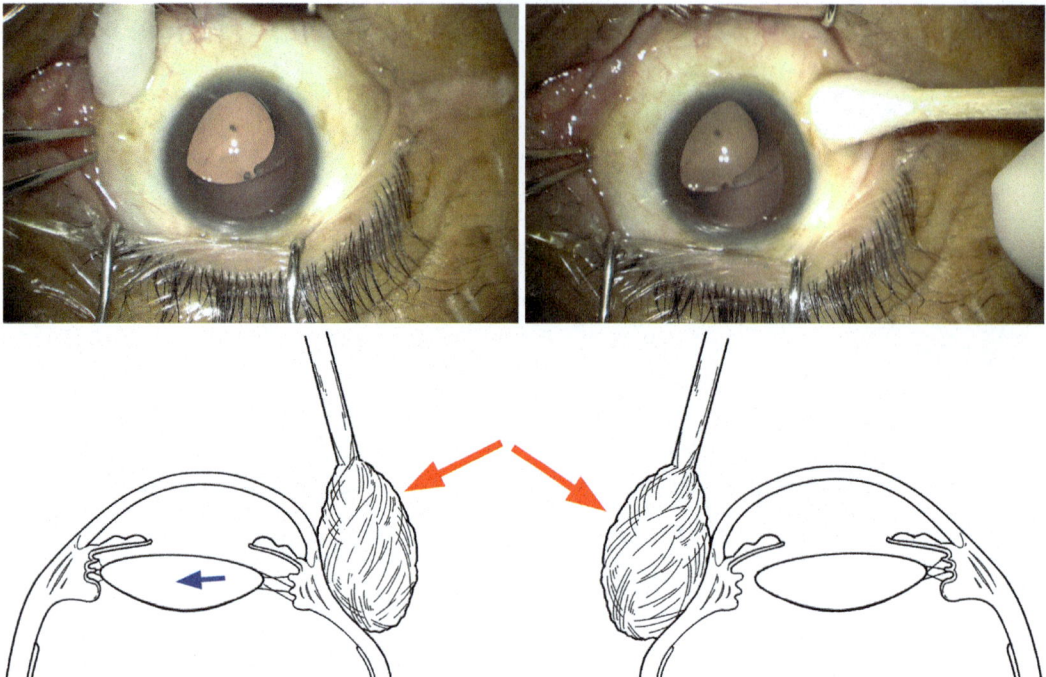

Fig. 11.2 Attachment of IOL is checked by pressing the globe (*Top Left*, *Bottom Left*). There is no IOL movement when press the detached quadrant (*Top Right*, *Bottom Right*)

length over than 12.5 mm and angulation of 5 degrees or more), I prefer to perform "one point scleral fixation" [1]. Choosing the suitable surgical procedure is dependent on the type of the IOL in the eye, amount and location of the zonular detachment.

Surgery 1. (Subluxated IOL Fixation)

1 mm corneal incision is made 90 degrees apart from the planned scleral fixation site. Conjunctival peritomies are created 180 degrees apart where the IOL haptic will be sutured. A long curved needle (PC-7 (Alcon, Fort Worth, Tex) or CTC-6 (Ethicon, Cornelia, Ga)) with 10–0 propylene suture is used to enter the eye perpendicular to the sclera and 1.5 mm posterior from the limbus, then passed under the haptic in anterior chamber. Rotate the long curved needle tip towards anterior chamber. 27G needle is passed through the corneal incision then is docked to the long curved needle. Withdraw the 27G needle and docked long curved needle together outside the eye

(Fig. 11.3). Detach 27G needle. Long curved needle is reintroduced again and pass it behind the iris, in front of the IOL haptic toward iris root. Exit the eye at least 1 mm closer towards the limbus than the previous ab interno passage (Fig. 11.4). The same procedure is used for the other haptic 180 degree apart when indicated.

Be sure not to catch corneal lip during passage of the long curved needle. Suture is tied and suture knot is rotated inward (Fig. 11.5). It is important not to cause severe tension to the remaining zonules that might cause secondary IOL dislocation due to loss of remaining zonules. Conjunctival incision is closed with 10-0 Nylon sutures.

Surgery 2. (Aphakia Correction, ab Externo) [2]

Half-thickness scleral flaps are fashioned in triangular shape 180 degrees apart. To avoid damaging long ciliary nerve and artery, the best to spare 3 and 9 o'clock position when making scleral flaps. The long, straight solid needle is

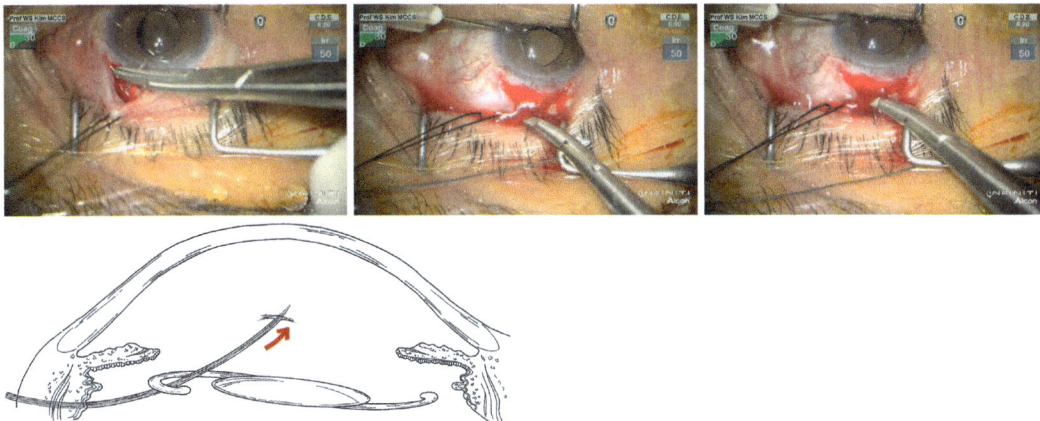

Fig. 11.3 A long curved needle is used to enter the eye perpendicular to the sclera (*Top Left*, *Bottom*). 27G needle is passed through the corneal incision (*Top Middle*). Withdraw the 27G needle and docked long curved needle together outside the eye (*Top Left*)

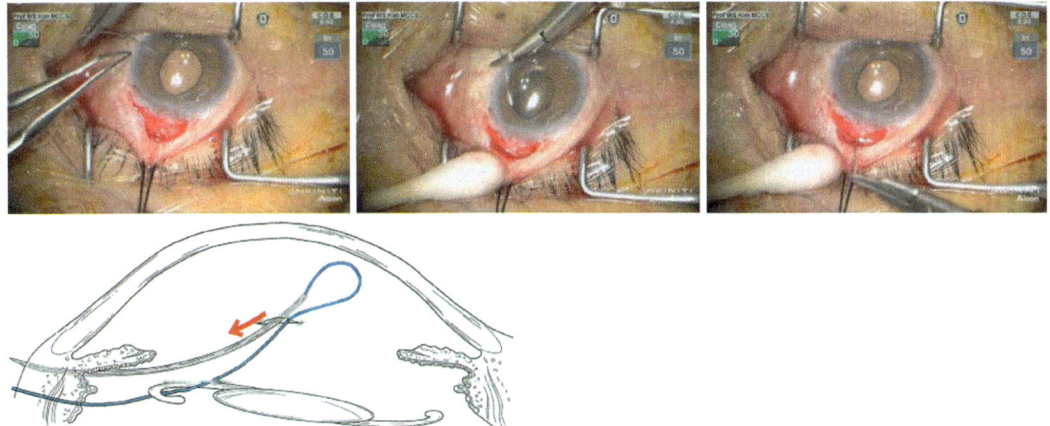

Fig. 11.4 Long curved needle is reintroduced again and pass it behind the iris, in front of the IOL haptic toward iris root (*Top Left*, *Bottom*). Exit the eye at least 1 mm closer towards the limbus than the previous ab interno passage (*Top Middle*, *Top Right*)

passed through the sclera approximately 1.5 mm posterior to the limbus. A second 27G needle is passed from the opposite side of the eye 1.5 mm posterior to the limbus.

Straight needle is "docked" to the tip of the hollow needle. After docking, the needles are withdrawn together towards the second needle's entry. A hook is used to pull the suture out through a limbal incision on superior quadrant so that it can be tied to the intraocular lens. After the IOL is placed into position, the scleral sutures must be anchored to the sclera.

Surgery 3. (Aphakia Correction, ab Interno)

Half-thickness scleral flaps are made as mentioned at surgery 2. Corneal incision is preferably made on the temporal quadrant between scleral flaps. First, a long curved needle (PC-7 (Alcon, Fort Worth, Tex) or CTC-6 (Ethicon, Cornelia, Ga)) is passed through the corneal incision, then under the iris aiming for the inferior ciliary sulcus. Location of the needle tip can be detected by indenting the sclera outward with the needle tip. If the needle tip is located too

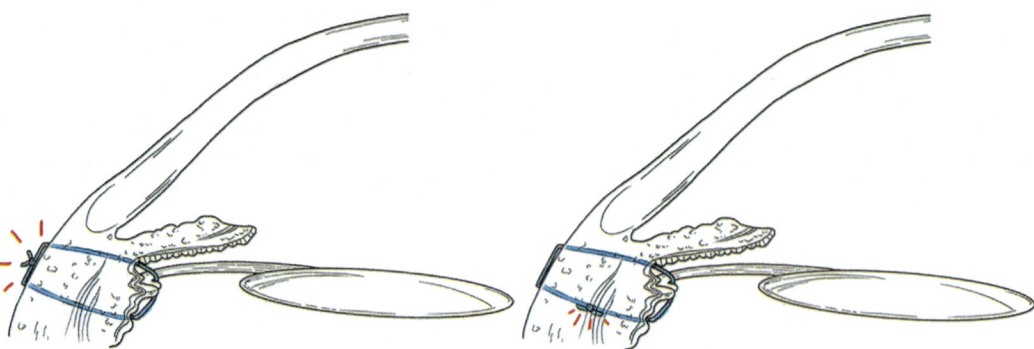

Fig. 11.5 Suture is tied and suture knot is rotated inward

anterior, iris dragging occurs. By moving the needle tip posteriorly from the iris root, needle can detect the recess present before rough ciliary body. Exit the needle through sclera once ciliary sulcus is found. One end of the IOL haptic is tied to the end of the long curved needle. IOL is folded and introduced into the eye leaving the trail haptic outside the eye. Trail haptic is also tied to second long curved needle and placed into the anterior chamber. Needle tip of the second long curved needle also fixated as mentioned for the first long curved needle.

After exiting the eye under the previously dissected scleral flaps, the sutures are tied, securing the intraocular lens into position. Appropriate suture tension is important to avoid lens decentration

Postoperative Considerations

> **Postoperative Medication**
>
> – Topical broad spectrum antibiotic: (Levofloxacin 0.5% [Cravit®, Santen, Japan] or Moxifloxacin 0.5% [Vigamox®, Alcon, USA] qid)
> – Topical steroids: (Prednisolone acetate 1% [Pred forte® , Allergan, USA] qid)
> – Topical NSAIDs: (Bromfenac [Bronuck®, Taejoon pharm., Korea] bid or Flurbiprofen sodium 0.03% [Flurbiprofen®, Basch&Lomb, USA] qid)

> – May require treatment of increased intraocular pressure: Dorzolamide/timolol [Cosopt®, Santen, Japan] bid, Brimonidine tartrate 0.1 % [Alphagan-P®, Allergan, USA] bid, Carbonic anhydrase inhibitor, acetazolamide [Acetazol®, Hanlim pharm., Korea]

Complications

After scleral suture of IOLs serious complications such as retinal detachment, hemorrhagic choroidal detachment, PBK, and later lens dislocation have been reported.

Persistent CME, glaucoma, uveitis, hyphema and vitreous hemorrhages, lens tilt or decentration are more frequent complications after scleral suture of IOLs. Patients are better tolerated with IOLs with large optics, because occurrence of lens decentration is frequent.

Erosions of the sutures through the conjunctiva are also common and they should be treated with grafting to avoid suture related endophthalmitis (sclera, pericardium, tendon, caruncle…).

IOL Dislocation and Iris Fixation of IOL

Usage of single piece acrylic IOL has been increased a lot. Most of the pseudophakic eyes these days were implanted with acrylic IOLs and so are most of the the eyes with dislocated IOLs in our practice.

Preoperative Considerations

Positions of the IOL, movability of the IOL should be evaluated before the surgery.

Surgery

With dilated pupil, side port 1 mm corneal incisions are made on 12 o'clock position. Incisions on 3 and 9 o'clock positions are placed on midperipheral location while that on 12 o'clock position is placed on limbus.

Cohesive viscoelasic is introduced into anterior chamber. Subluxated IOL is delivered to anterior chamber using Sinskey hook (Fig. 11.6). While round spatula is placed behind the IOL optic, IOL haptics are rotated and pushed behind the iris (Fig. 11.7). With IOL optic stays above the iris plane, miotics is injected into the anterior chamber (Fig. 11.8). Wait until IOL optic is captured by the iris. With the IOL optic kept above the iris plane with round spatula or long needle, visualization of IOL haptic becomes prominent, a long curved needle is passes though the surface of the cornea then through the iris surface 1 clock hour apart close to pupillary ruff then pass behind the IOL haptic, then penetrate the iris stroma again on other side of the IOL haptic. Then, the needle is drawn outside of the eye. Same procedure is performed for the other loop of the IOL haptic (Fig. 11.9).

Fixation sutures placed peripheral iris tends to cheese-wire iris stromal tissue, we preferred to place fixation sutures over peripheral part of the pupillary sphincter muscle in order not to lose the fixation sutures.

Corneal stab incisions made on closed to the location of the iris fixation sutures (Fig. 11.10). A hook, made with 20G needle whose tip bented towards the bevel, introduced through the corneal incision to catch the loose ends of the fixation sutures. Both ends of the sutures are withdrawn and tied securely (Fig. 11.11). Same procedure is performed for both haptics. Any dragged vitreous is cut with scissors or vitrector. Viscoelastic is removed with bimanual I&A or by injecting BSS. Always be ready to remove any vitreous present in anterior chamber to minimize the risk of vitreous incarceration.

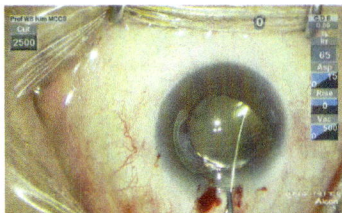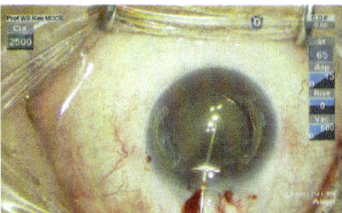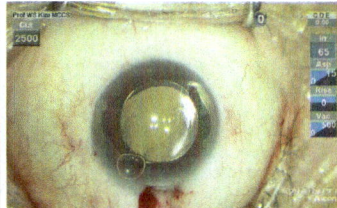

Fig. 11.6 Subluxated IOL is delivered to anterior chamber using Sinskey hook

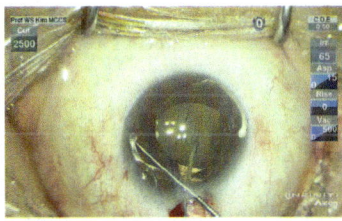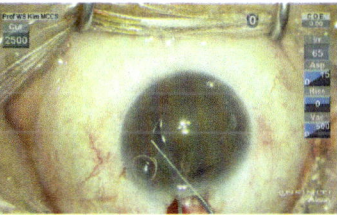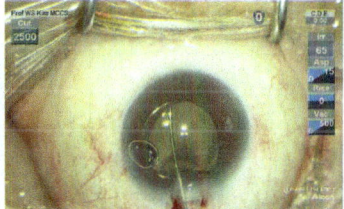

Fig. 11.7 While round spatula is placed behind the IOL optic, IOL haptics are rotated and pushed behind the iris

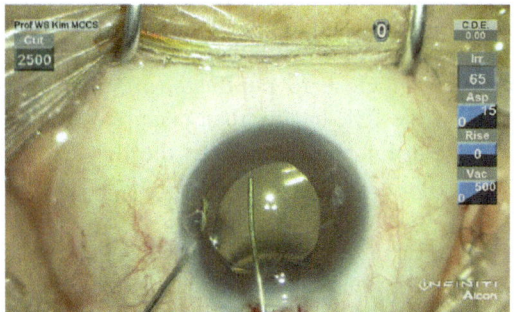

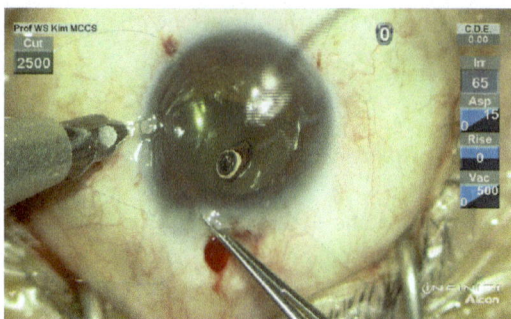

Fig. 11.8 With IOL optic stays above the iris plane, miotics is injected into the anterior chamber

Fig. 11.10 Corneal stab incisions made on closed to the location of the iris fixation sutures

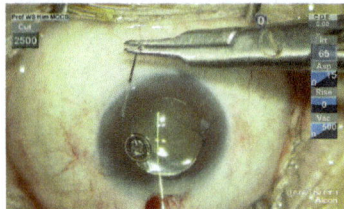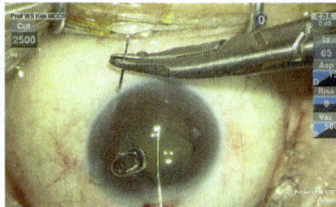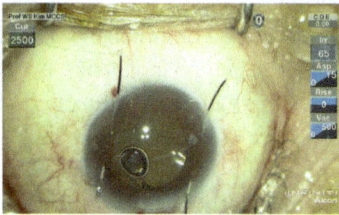

Fig. 11.9 Long curved needle is passed though the surface of cornea then passed behind the IOL haptic (*Left*, *Middle*). Same procedure is performed for the other loop of the IOL haptic (*Left*).

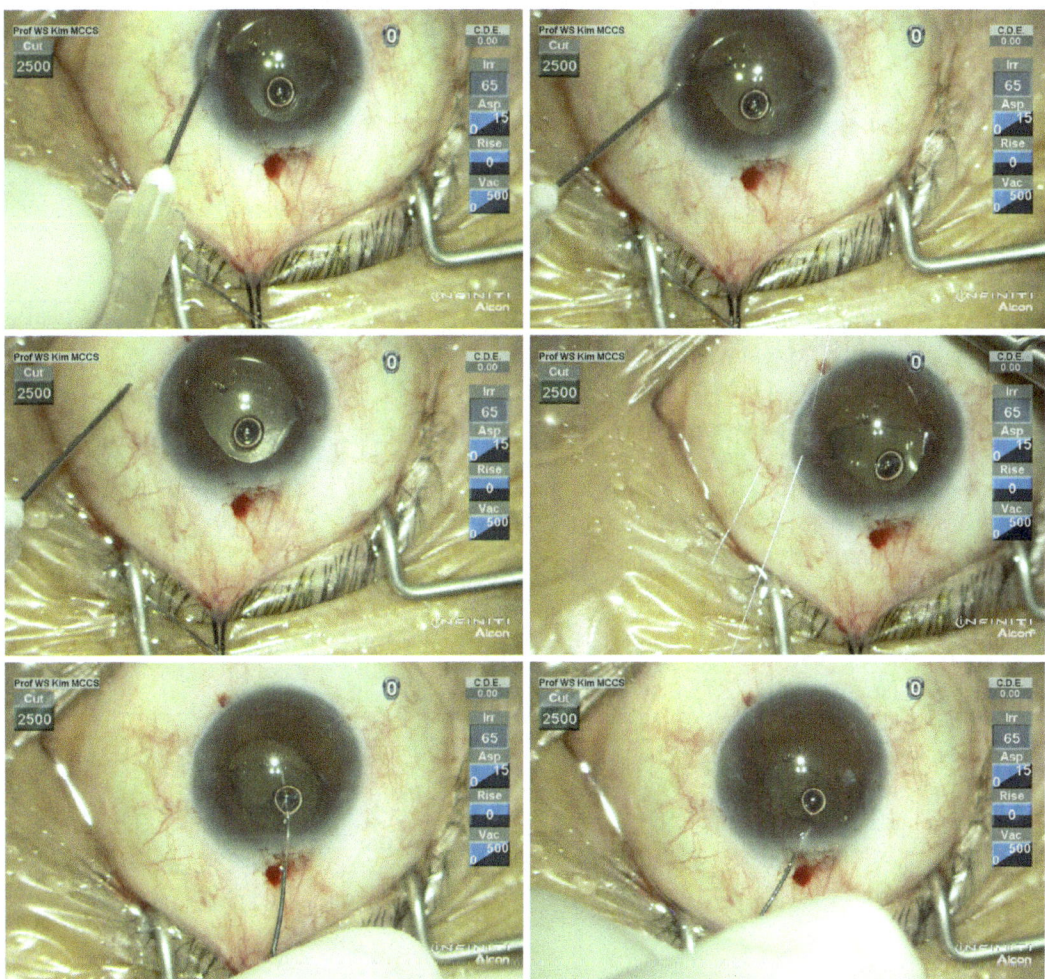

Fig. 11.11 A hook, made with 20G needle whose tip bented towards the bevel, introduced through the corneal incision to catch the loose ends of the fixation sutures (*Top Left*, *Top Right*). Both ends of the sutures are withdrawn and tied securely (*Middle Left*, *Middle Right*). Captured IOL is repositioned (*Bottom Left*, *Bottom Right*)

Postoperative Considerations

Vitreous incarceration is common and laser vitreolysis can be considered.

Postoperative Medication

- Topical broad spectrum antibiotic: (Levofloxacin 0.5% [Cravit®, Santen, Japan] or Moxifloxacin 0.5% [Vigamox®, Alcon, USA] qid)
- Topical steroids: (Prednisolone acetate 1% [Pred forte®, Allergan, USA] qid)
- Topical NSAIDs: (Bromfenac [Bronuck®, Taejoon pharm., Korea] bid or Flurbiprofen sodium 0.03% [Flurbiprofen®, Basch&Lomb, USA] qid)
- May require treatment of increased intraocular pressure: Dorzolamide/timolol [Cosopt®, Santen, Japan] bid, Brimonidine tartrate 0.1% [Alphagan-P®, Allergan, USA] bid, Carbonic anhydrase inhibitor, acetazolamide [Acetazol®, Hanlim pharm., Korea]

Complication (Table 11.1)

Uveitis

Iris-sutued lenses may cause more inflammation as a result of irritation of uveal tissue because of suspension of the relatively heavy IOL from the iris

Table 11.1 Complications of scleral and iris fixation [3]

	Scleral fixation group (N=44 eyes)	Iris fixation group (N=35 eyes)	p
Intraocular bleeding, n (%)	2 (4.5%)	0 (0%)	.50
Endothelial cell loss (mean±SD, %)	10.9±9.2	12.7±8.7	.16
AC cell grade at POD 1 (mean±SD)	0.9±1.1	1.7±0.7	.001
AC flare grade at POD 3 (mean±SD)	0.6±0.8	1.0±1.3	.26
Clinical CME, n (%)	0 (0%)	1 (2.9%)	.44
Retinal detachment, n (%)	1 (2.3%)	0 (0%)	1.00
Recurrence of IOL dislocation, n (%)	6 (13.6%)	6 (17.1%)	.67
Interval (mean±SD, mo)	10.0+9.3	1.7+0.7	.031
Early recurrence (<3 months)	3	6	.046

References

1. Kanigowska K, Grałek M. Posterior chamber intraocular lens implantation with one-point scleral fixation in children in long time observation. Klin Oczna. 2011;113:19–21.
2. Mittelviefhaus H, Wiek J. A refined technique of transscleral suture fixation of posterior chamber lenses developed for cases of complicated cataract surgery with vitreous loss. Ophthalmic Surg. 1993;24:698–701.
3. Kim KH, Kim WS. Comparison of clinical outcomes of iris fixation and scleral fixation as treatment for intraocular lens dislocation. Am J Ophthalmol. 2015;160:463–9.

High myopia, generally defined as an axial length longer than 26.0 mm or myopia greater than −6.0 diopters (D), is a commonly encountered comorbidity in cataract patients. The prevalence of high myopia in the general population has been reported to range from 2 to 5 %, but it may be as high as 10–21 % especially in ethnic Asians and younger persons [1–5]. In addition, high myopia is strongly associated with increased rates of nuclear and posterior subcapsular cataract [6, 7].

Preoperative Considerations

High myopia carries a risk of other ocular comorbidities, such as open angle glaucoma, chorioretinal atrophy, foveomacular schisis and retinal detachment [8]. As these comorbidities can affect postoperative visual outcomes, careful and thorough preoperative examinations of highly myopic patients, and counseling of these patients on expected outcomes and complications, are important. Retinal examinations, including dilated fundoscopy and optical coherence tomography, are required to assess retinal pathologies such as peripheral retinal tear and maculopathy, as patients with the former condition are at risk for retinal detachment and those with the latter pathology show higher rates of failure to achieve good postoperative vision [9, 10]. Although the risk of retinal detachment after cataract surgery may be related to increases in axial length and anterior chamber depth [10], the incidence of retinal detachment after cataract surgery in highly myopic patients did not differ significantly from the incidence of pseudophakic or idiopathic retinal detachment in mildly to moderately myopic patients [11]. Highly myopic patients seem to benefit from cataract surgery for refractive correction, as long as they are examined preoperatively and receive appropriate prophylaxis for retinal pathology.

High myopia may also affect surgical outcomes indirectly. Posterior staphyloma may induce measurement errors, especially when using ultrasound to measure axial length, resulting in undesirable refractive outcomes. Although its accuracy may be lower in eyes with axial length greater than 30 mm [12], optical biometry using partial coherence laser interferometry may produce more accurate and reproducible results in highly myopic patients [13], because indentation of the cornea could be avoided and patient fixation on the measuring beam may prevent eccentric measurement on the staphyloma. Commonly used standard third generation intraocular lens (IOL) calculation formulas with standard IOL constants could also lead to unexpected postoperative hyperopia in eyes of greater axial length [14–16]. These problems have been addressed by the introduction of new formulas, such as the Holladay 2, Olsen and Barrett Universal II formulas [15, 17, 18]. In using A constants from the IOL manufacturer, the Haigis formula was shown to produce the least mean absolute error, followed in order by the SRK/T,

Holladay 2, Holladay 1 and Hoffer Q formulas [16]. Although the Haigis formula was the most accurate in the total population of studied eyes, the SRK/T formula was the most accurate in eyes of axial length 27.0–29.07 mm [16]. This problem may also be addressed by using specific IOL constants for eyes of greater axial length, because there is a potential problem in calculating IOL power for eyes with extreme myopia in the vicinity of the transition between plus-power and minus-power IOLs [19, 20]. Changes in the sign of IOL power have been associated with changes in IOL geometry, altering the position of the principal planes from the anterior to the posterior side of the IOL, or vice versa. Because the principal plane position is associated with the effective lens position, a change in principal plane position would have a direct effect on IOL constants, which are directly associated with effective lens positions. Therefore, different IOL constants should be applied to plus and minus IOLs. If existing constants for plus IOLs are also used for minus IOLs, hyperopic refractive errors can occur, which worsen with increasing axial length [20]. In addition to using a specific IOL constant, optimization of axial length may improve prediction accuracy [21]. Equations that may optimize axial length include: Holladay 1 optimized axial length $= 0.8814 \times$ IOLMaster axial length $+ 2.8701$; Haigis optimized axial length $= 0.9621 \times$ IOLMaster axial length $+ 0.6763$; SRK/T optimized axial length $= 0.8981 \times$ IOLMaster axial length $+ 2.5637$; and Hoffer Q optimized axial length $= 0.8776 \times$ IOLMaster axial length $+ 2.9269$ [21]. Results comparing the accuracy of these formulas indicate that the SRK/T formula, the Haigis formula using the framework of the User Group for Laser Interference Biometry project to optimize constants for optical biometry, and the Barrett Universal II, Holladay 2, and Olsen formulas provide the most predictable outcomes with an IOL power of 6.0 D and higher for eyes of axial length greater than 26.0 mm. The Holladay 1 and Haigis formulas with axial length adjustment, and the Barrett Universal II formula, were most accurate in predicting refraction for IOL power less than 6.0 D [15].

When using common IOL formulas with each manufacturer's optical constants and IOLMaster [16] and aiming for emmetropia, targeting a postoperative refraction of −0.5 to −2.0 D may be reasonable. As shown by the relationships between mean absolute errors and axial length, target refractions of −0.25 D to −0.75 D, −0.5 D to −1.00 D, and −1.00 D to −1.75 D were reasonable for eyes with axial lengths of 27–29 mm, 29–30 mm, and greater than 30 mm, respectively [16].

Although multifocal IOLs can be implanted into highly myopic eyes, there is a possibility of progressive change in axial length and resultant refractive error, because axial length was found to continue to increase in 30 % of highly myopic eyes [22]. In addition, multifocal IOLs should be avoided in highly myopic eyes with any retinal comorbidity, even if the latter is of mild severity, because myopic maculopathy tends to progress in approximately 40 % of highly myopic eyes [23].

Intraoperative Considerations

Highly myopic eyes are among the most challenging on which to perform cataract surgery. Eyes with high myopia often have thinly stretched zonules and underdeveloped ciliary bodies. Therefore, infusion into the anterior chamber during phacoemulsification may lead to lens-iris diaphragm retropulsion syndrome (LIDRS), which is characterized by marked deepening and fluctuation of the anterior chamber, posterior iris bowing, pupil dilation, and significant discomfort (Fig. 12.1) [24, 25]. Because topical anesthesia alone cannot prevent all pain and discomfort, administration of preservative-free 1 % lidocaine hydrochloride into the capsular bag during hydrodissection may improve intraoperative comfort. [26] In addition, lowering the bottle height in conjunction with commensurate reductions in the vacuum and flow rate during phacoemulsification may prevent LIDRS and patient discomfort. Meticulous manipulation of a foot pedal to slowly increase infusion pressure when inserting the hand-pieces for phacoemulsification

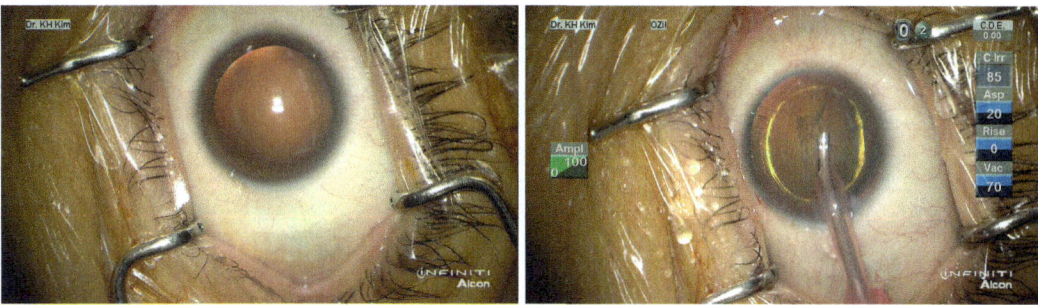

Fig. 12.1 (*Left*) The anterior chamber is filled with ophthalmic viscosurgical devices and the iris is dilated, however, (*Right*) the insertion of the phacoemulsification tip and the concommitant irrigation lead to marked deepening of the anterior chamber and further dilation of the pupil with posterior bowing of the iris

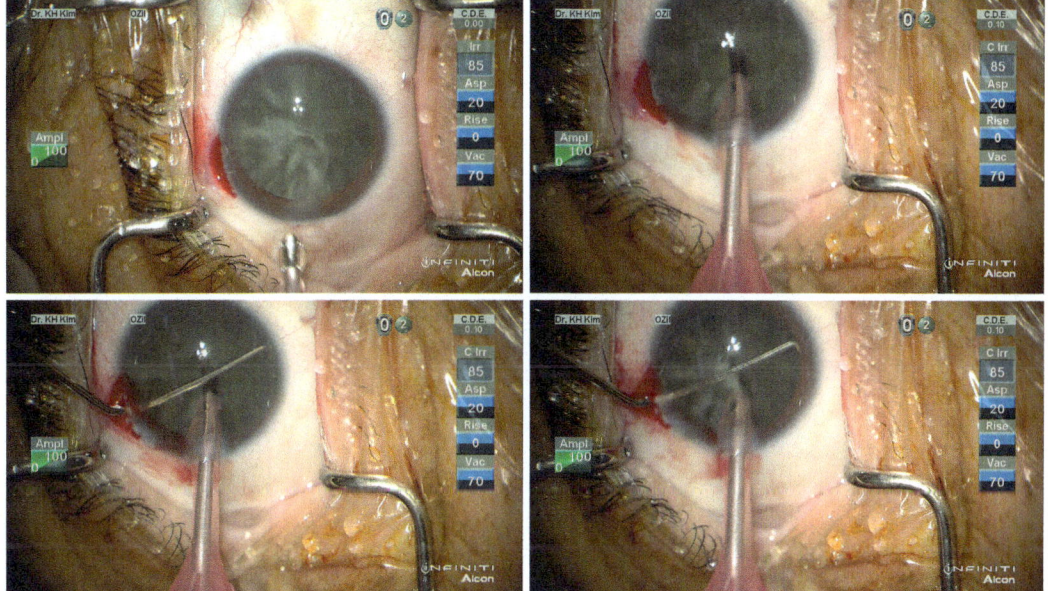

Fig. 12.2 (*Top*, *Left*) The anterior chamber is filled with ophthalmic viscosurgical devices and the iris is dilated, however, (*Top*, *Right*) the insertion of the phacoemulsification tip and the concommitant irrigation lead to marked deepening of the anterior chamber and further dilation of the pupil with posterior bowing of the iris. (*Bottom*, *Left*) A second instrument can be used to immediately lift the iris margin, equalizing pressure between the anterior and posterior chambers, (*Bottom*, *Right*) relieving patient discomfort and reversing this phenomenon

may also stabilize the anterior chamber and prevent LIDRS. If LIDRS occurs despite these techniques, a second instrument can be used to immediately lift the iris margin, equalizing pressure between the anterior and posterior chambers, relieving patient discomfort and reversing LIDRS (Figs. 12.2 and 12.3) [27].

The size of the capsular bag and the horizontal diameter between the sulci are often proportionately wider in eyes with greater axial length than in normal eyes [28]. Hence, when implanting IOLs in eyes with greater axial length, IOLs of greater optical diameter and total length are advantageous as they reduce the likelihood of IOL instability due to lower equatorial friction [29], which can lead to serious complications such as uveitis-glaucoma-hemorrhage syndrome. This issue is of particular importance when IOLs are implanted in the sulcus of eyes of greater axial length. Refractive outcomes

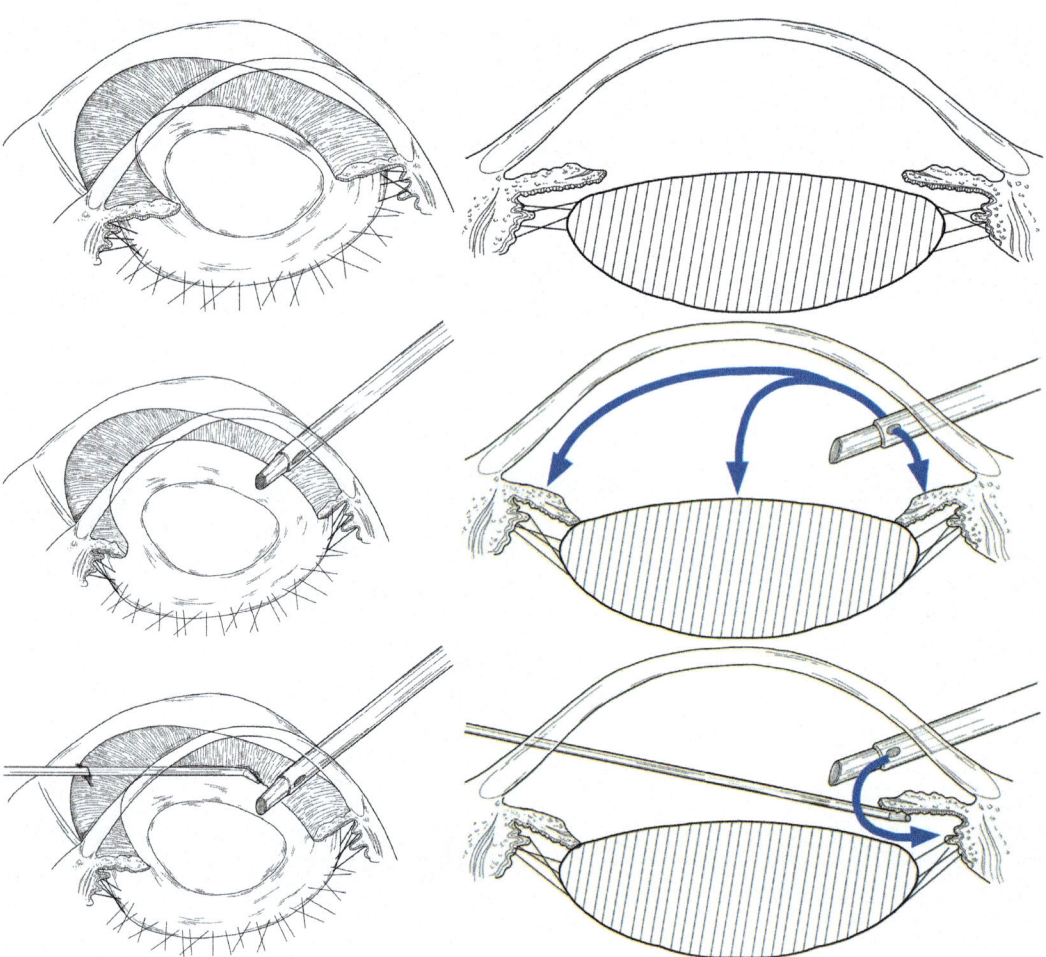

Fig. 12.3 (*Top Left* and *Right*) In eyes with thinly stretched zonules and underdeveloped ciliary bodies, (*Center Left* and *Right*) an infusion into the anterior chamber may deepen the anterior chamber and push iris posteriorly, causing marked pupillary dilation and patient's discomfort. (*Bottom Left* and *Right*) This phenomenon could be reversed after pressure equalization between anterior and posterior chamber by lifting iris margin for the irrigation flow to be entered into the posterior chamber between the iris and lens capsule

following implantation of toric IOLs into eyes of greater axial length may be more vulnerable to rotational instability than into eyes with normal axial length. Therefore, when implanting toric IOLs into the former, designs with greater total length should be selected. In addition, a capsular tension ring (CTR) may stabilize the capsular bag and prevent rotation of the IOL, because it theoretically enforces symmetry on the bag, stretching its equator, flattening its anterior–posterior axis, increasing friction on the IOL haptics and enhancing stability [30]. In this situation, it is not necessary to modify IOL

power calculations because CTRs do not have consistent effects on refractive outcomes, even in highly myopic eyes [31]. Zero-powered IOLs may be necessary for eyes of axial length between 31 and 32 mm, although the need for such IOLs depends on the combination of axial length and corneal radii of curvature and not on axial length alone [20]. Zero-powered IOLs may be more advantageous than planned aphakia, because these IOLs may provide a barrier between the vitreous cavity and the anterior chamber, preventing vitreous prolapse and further corneal and retinal morbidities. However, zero-powered IOLs could also produce a hyperopic error, typically around 0.25 D, as a result of beam-widening effects [20].

Postoperative Considerations

Despite advances in biometry and IOL power calculations, cataract patients with high myopia remain at risk for clinically significant ametropia. Excimer laser surgery, such as photorefractive keratectomy or laser in situ keratomileusis, can correct ametropia after cataract surgery [32, 33]. However, postoperative ametropia in highly myopic eyes may be large and hyperopic rather than myopic, with hyperopia less effectively corrected by excimer based corneal surgery. In these eyes, residual refractive error may be corrected by IOL exchange or piggyback IOL. The implantation of a secondary piggyback IOL into the ciliary sulcus, while leaving the original IOL in place, has been shown to be effective and safe for a pseudophakic refractive surprise and is believed to be more precise than IOL exchange, because piggyback IOL surgery avoids the need to determine the cause of the error [34]. Furthermore, double IOLs can significantly improve axial modulation function, which translates clinically into better contrast sensitivity in highly hyperopic eyes [35]. The use of multifocal IOLs is especially limited in highly myopic patients, due to the unavailability of negatively powered multifocal IOLs. However, implantation of a secondary piggyback IOL with a refractive multifocal design may achieve good near-intermediate visual acuity and spectacle independence, especially in highly myopic eyes with good near visual acuity. In addition, a secondary piggyback IOL can correct residual refractive errors remaining after implantation of a monofocal IOL, as the implanted lens can be tolerated monocularly [36].

References

1. Pan CW, Klein BE, Cotch MF, et al. Racial variations in the prevalence of refractive errors in the United States: the multi-ethnic study of atherosclerosis. Am J Ophthalmol. 2013;155:1129–38.e1.

2. McCarty CA, Livingston PM, Taylor HR. Prevalence of myopia in adults: implications for refractive surgeons. J Refract Surg (Thorofare, NJ: 1995). 1997;13:229–34.

3. Hyman L. Myopic and hyperopic refractive error in adults: an overview. Ophthalmic Epidemiol. 2007;14:192–7.

4. Wong TY, Foster PJ, Hee J, et al. Prevalence and risk factors for refractive errors in adult Chinese in Singapore. Invest Ophthalmol Vis Sci. 2000;41:2486–94.

5. Lin LL, Shih YF, Hsiao CK, Chen CJ. Prevalence of myopia in Taiwanese schoolchildren: 1983 to 2000. Ann Acad Med Singapore. 2004;33:27–33.

6. Kanthan GL, Mitchell P, Rochtchina E, Cumming RG, Wang JJ. Myopia and the long-term incidence of cataract and cataract surgery: the Blue Mountains Eye Study. Clin Experiment Ophthalmol. 2014;42:347–53.

7. Pan CW, Boey PY, Cheng CY, et al. Myopia, axial length, and age-related cataract: the Singapore Malay eye study. Invest Ophthalmol Vis Sci. 2013;54:4498–502.

8. Chong EW, Mehta JS. High myopia and cataract surgery. Curr Opin Ophthalmol. 2015.

9. Tsai CY, Chang TJ, Kuo LL, Chou P, Woung LC. Visual outcomes and associated risk factors of cataract surgeries in highly myopic Taiwanese. Ophthalmologica J Int D'ophtalmologie Int J Ophthalmol Zeitschrift fur Augenheilkunde. 2008;222:130–5.

10. Bhagwandien AC, Cheng YY, Wolfs RC, van Meurs JC, Luyten GP. Relationship between retinal detachment and biometry in 4262 cataractous eyes. Ophthalmology. 2006;113:643–9.

11. Neuhann IM, Neuhann TF, Heimann H, Schmickler S, Gerl RH, Foerster MH. Retinal detachment after phacoemulsification in high myopia: analysis of 2356 cases. J Cataract Refract Surg. 2008;34:1644–57.

12. Roessler GF, Dietlein TS, Plange N, et al. Accuracy of intraocular lens power calculation using partial coherence interferometry in patients with high myopia. Ophthalmic Physiol Opt J B Coll Ophthalmic Opticians Optometrists. 2012;32:228–33.

13. Findl O, Drexler W, Menapace R, Heinzl H, Hitzenberger CK, Fercher AF. Improved prediction of intraocular lens power using partial coherence interferometry. J Cataract Refract Surg. 2001;27:861–7.

14. Zaldivar R, Shultz MC, Davidorf JM, Holladay JT. Intraocular lens power calculations in patients with extreme myopia. J Cataract Refract Surg. 2000;26:668–74.

15. Abulafia A, Barrett GD, Rotenberg M, et al. Intraocular lens power calculation for eyes with an axial length greater than 26.0 mm: comparison of formulas and methods. J Cataract Refract Surg. 2015;41:548–56.

16. Bang S, Edell E, Yu Q, Pratzer K, Stark W. Accuracy of intraocular lens calculations using the IOLMaster

in eyes with long axial length and a comparison of various formulas. Ophthalmology. 2011;118:503–6.

17. Olsen T. Prediction of the effective postoperative (intraocular lens) anterior chamber depth. J Cataract Refract Surg. 2006;32:419–24.

18. Barrett GD. An improved universal theoretical formula for intraocular lens power prediction. J Cataract Refract Surg. 1993;19:713–20.

19. Petermeier K, Gekeler F, Messias A, Spitzer MS, Haigis W, Szurman P. Intraocular lens power calculation and optimized constants for highly myopic eyes. J Cataract Refract Surg. 2009;35:1575–81.

20. Haigis W. Intraocular lens calculation in extreme myopia. J Cataract Refract Surg. 2009;35:906–11.

21. Wang L, Shirayama M, Ma XJ, Kohnen T, Koch DD. Optimizing intraocular lens power calculations in eyes with axial lengths above 25.0 mm. J Cataract Refract Surg. 2011;37:2018–27.

22. Saka N, Ohno-Matsui K, Shimada N, et al. Long-term changes in axial length in adult eyes with pathologic myopia. Am J Ophthalmol. 2010;150:562–8.e1.

23. Hayashi K, Ohno-Matsui K, Shimada N, et al. Long-term pattern of progression of myopic maculopathy: a natural history study. Ophthalmology. 2010;117:1595–611, 1611.e1–4.

24. Wilbrandt HR, Wilbrandt TH. Pathogenesis and management of the lens-iris diaphragm retropulsion syndrome during phacoemulsification. J Cataract Refract Surg. 1994;20:48–53.

25. Zauberman H. Extreme deepening of the anterior chamber during phacoemulsification. Ophthalmic Surg. 1992;23:555–6.

26. Lofoco G, Ciucci F, Bardocci A, et al. Efficacy of topical plus intracameral anesthesia for cataract surgery in high myopia: randomized controlled trial. J Cataract Refract Surg. 2008;34:1664–8.

27. Cheung CM, Hero M. Stabilization of anterior chamber depth during phacoemulsification cataract surgery

in vitrectomized eyes. J Cataract Refract Surg. 2005;31:2055–7.

28. Lim SJ, Kang SJ, Kim HB, Kurata Y, Sakabe I, Apple DJ. Analysis of zonular-free zone and lens size in relation to axial length of eye with age. J Cataract Refract Surg. 1998;24:390–6.

29. Chang DF. Early rotational stability of the longer Staar toric intraocular lens: fifty consecutive cases. J Cataract Refract Surg. 2003;29:935–40.

30. Sagiv O, Sachs D. Rotation stability of a toric intraocular lens with a second capsular tension ring. J Cataract Refract Surg. 2015;41:1098–9.

31. Schild AM, Rosentreter A, Hellmich M, Lappas A, Dinslage S, Dietlein TS. Effect of a capsular tension ring on refractive outcomes in eyes with high myopia. J Cataract Refract Surg. 2010;36:2087–93.

32. Kuo IC, O'Brien TP, Broman AT, Ghajarnia M, Jabbur NS. Excimer laser surgery for correction of ametropia after cataract surgery. J Cataract Refract Surg. 2005;31:2104–10.

33. Kim P, Briganti EM, Sutton GL, Lawless MA, Rogers CM, Hodge C. Laser in situ keratomileusis for refractive error after cataract surgery. J Cataract Refract Surg. 2005;31:979–86.

34. El Awady HE, Ghanem AA. Secondary piggyback implantation versus IOL exchange for symptomatic pseudophakic residual ametropia. Graefe's Arch Clin Exp Ophthalmol = Albrecht von Graefes Archiv fur klinische und experimentelle Ophthalmologie. 2013;251:1861–6.

35. Hull CC, Liu CS, Sciscio A. Image quality in polypseudophakia for extremely short eyes. Br J Ophthalmol. 1999;83:656–63.

36. Huerva V. Piggyback multifocal IOLs for a hyperopic-presbyopic surprise after cataract surgery in high myopic patients. Cont Lens Anterior Eye J B Contact Lens Association. 2014;37:57–9.

Eyes smaller than normal (axial length less than 20.5 mm) can be classified into two categories according to anterior chamber depth: those with microphthalmos (short anterior chamber depth) and those with high axial hyperopia (normal anterior chamber depth) [1]. Eyes with short anterior chamber depth and normal axial length are classified as having relative anterior microphthalmos (Fig. 13.1) [2]. Depending on the presence or absence of an accompanying anatomic malformation in the anterior or posterior segment of the eye, eyes with microphthalmos may be subdivided further into those with simple microphthalmos (or nanophthalmos) and complex microphthalmos [3]. In the latter, microphthalmos is accompanied by anatomic malformations, including chorioretinal colobomas, persistent hyperplastic primary vitreous, and retinal dysplasia [3]. Phacoemulsification of these eyes and implantation of intraocular lenses (IOLs) are challenging, with high risks of intraoperative and postoperative complications such as zonular dehiscence, severe uveitis, uveal effusion, cystoid macular edema and aqueous misdirection. Furthermore, the risk of complications increases in proportion to the reduction in axial length [4]. Recent developments in phacoemulsification and devices used for IOL implantation have overcome these challenges, resulting in satisfactory clinical outcomes [4–6].

Preoperative Considerations

The crystalline lens in eyes with microphthalmos is normal in volume, despite ocular volume being approximately two-thirds that of an average eye [1]. Crowding of the anterior segment by a disproportionately large crystalline lens results in a shallower anterior chamber and angle closure glaucoma [3]. The anterior chamber angle can also be closed by physical displacement of the peripheral iris by anteriorly rotated ciliary processes when annular ciliochoroidal effusion and ciliary body detachment are present [7]. Response to medical treatment is poor and miotics may even worsen this condition by relaxing the lens zonules in these patients. Laser iridotomy in the early stage of glaucoma can eliminate the pupillary block component before the occurrence of peripheral anterior synechia formation, but usually does not provide sufficient control of intraocular pressure. Laser iridoplasty can be performed if the anterior chamber remains appositionally closed after iridectomy [8]. If peripheral anterior synechia develops, glaucoma surgery may be required; however, the risk of complications is high [9]. Phacoemulsification of and IOL implantation into microphthalmic eyes can simultaneously manage both cataract and abnormal intraocular pressure, because cataract surgery can deepen the anterior chamber and widen the anterior chamber angle, reducing intraocular pressure [10]. In addition to improving

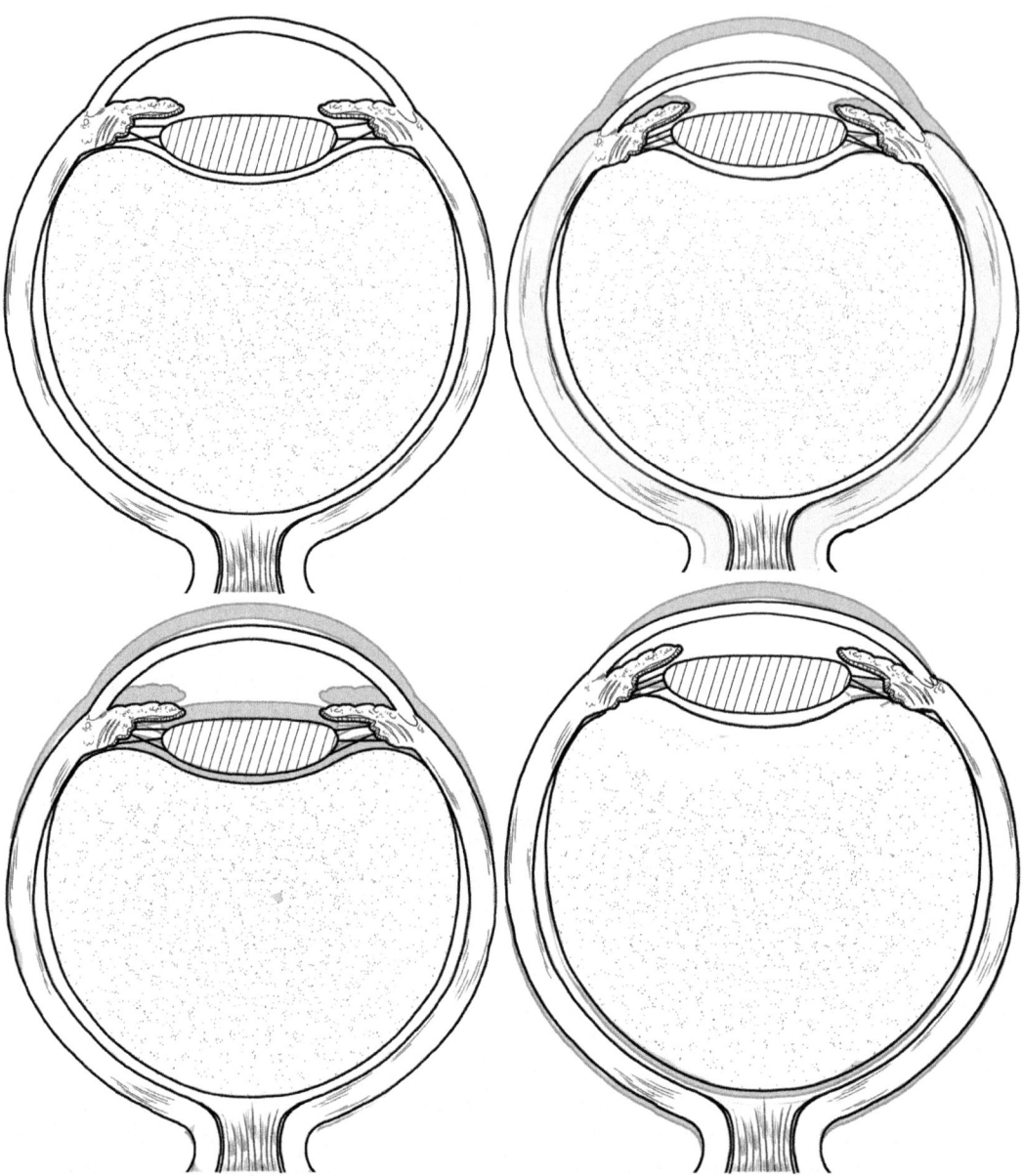

Fig. 13.1 (*Top, Left*) Compared to a normal eye, (*Top, Right*) an eye with microophthalmos shows shorter axial length and crowded anterior chamber with thickened scleral wall. (*Bottom, Left*) An eye with axial hyperopia is smaller than normal eye, but anterior chamber depth is not affected. (*Bottom, Right*) Eyes with short anterior chamber depth and normal axial length are classified as having relative anterior microphthalmos

intraocular pressure control rather than treating visually significant cataract, crystalline lens removal and IOL implantation may be useful in correcting hyperopia.

Complex microphthalmos may be accompanied by congenital or hereditary ocular pathologies, including Leber congenital amaurosis,

oculocutaneous albinism, retinal coloboma, congenital cataract, retinitis pigmentosa and corneal dystrophy [3, 5]. Visual outcomes in these eyes may be poorer than in eyes with microphthalmos unaccompanied by associated ocular diseases or with an acquired ocular pathology, such as chronic angle closure glaucoma, pseudoexfoliation syndrome or diabetic maculopathy [5]. Comorbidities should therefore be carefully evaluated to predict visual outcomes.

IOL power calculation in these extremely small eyes may be inaccurate. Because ultrasound waves travel faster through the lens than through the vitreous, ultrasound may underestimate axial length in microphthalmic eyes with relatively large crystalline lenses [3, 11]. In addition, errors in measuring axial length would have a greater effect on refractive outcomes because any errors in measurement would constitute a higher percent of axial length in these eyes [11]. Furthermore, IOL power calculating formulas that assume a fixed anterior chamber depth would result in much larger errors in calculation [3]. When using A constants from the manufacturer of the IOL, the Hoffer Q formula has been found to produce the least mean absolute error in eyes with axial length less than 22.0 mm (range 19.23–21.98 mm), followed by the Holladay 1 formula, with both significantly lower than SRK/T [12]. The mean absolute errors for all formulae, including SRK/T and Haigis, were significantly reduced by IOL constant adjustment; for example, using an A constant of 118.5 for the Akreos Adapt (Bausch & Lomb) rather than the constant of 118.0 provided by the IOL manufacturer. Another study of 608 eyes with axial length less than 22.0 mm found that the Hoffer Q had the lowest mean absolute error for axial lengths from 20.00 to 21.49 mm and that the Holladay 1 performed best for axial lengths from 21.00 to 21.49 mm [13]. However, as refractive predictability and postoperative outcomes were poorer in eyes with nanophthalmos than in normal eyes and those with relative anterior microphthalmos [14], patients with short axial length should be counselled preoperatively about the potential for poor refractive outcomes.

Intraoperative Considerations

Selection of anesthetic techniques is problematic in eyes with short axial length. Because of the risks of increased posterior pressure cause by regional blocks, such as peribulbar or retrobulbar anesthesia, topical anesthesia may be safer and preferred by some surgeons [14–16]. However, topical anesthesia would also not be satisfactory because of the potential for greater than normal intraocular manipulation. Therefore, some surgeons prefer peribulbar or retrobulbar anesthesia [5, 6, 10, 17, 18].

Eyes with microphthalmos and relative anterior microphthalmos are at higher risk for damage to the corneal endothelium during phacoemulsification and for resultant postoperative corneal edema due to the more crowded and shallower anterior chamber [2, 5, 6, 14, 19]. The anterior chamber in these eyes may be deepened by injection of an ophthalmic viscosurgical device (OVD) of dispersive type into the anterior chamber through the paracentesis. If this fails to deepen the anterior chamber, a limited pars plana vitrectomy with one port, removing a small amount of retro-lental vitreous (approximately 0.2–0.3 cc) with a 25-gauge high-speed cutter, may increase anterior chamber depth [20]. Preoperative administration of oral acetazolamide (500 mg) and intravenous 10 % mannitol (1 g/kg) may also reduce the risk of shallowing of the anterior chamber [6]. The risk of endothelial cell loss during phacoemulsification may be reduced by using a soft-shell technique, in which the endothelium is coated with a lower viscosity dispersive OVD followed by coating with a higher viscosity cohesive OVD for surgical maneuvers [21].

Posterior synechia and undulating pupil, which frequently accompany microphthalmos [3], may be successfully managed by gentle synechiolysis using a cyclodialysis spatula and several pupil dilating maneuvers, including intracameral mydriatics, pupillary membrane dissection and pupil expansion using OVD or iris hooks (see Chap. 4). If laser peripheral iridotomy has not been previously performed, peripheral iridectomy may prevent angle closure glaucoma after the cataract surgery in these microphthalmic eyes. However, although surgeons perform peripheral iridectomy for this purpose, a significant association between such surgery and reduced rates of angle closure glaucoma has yet to be demonstrated [6].

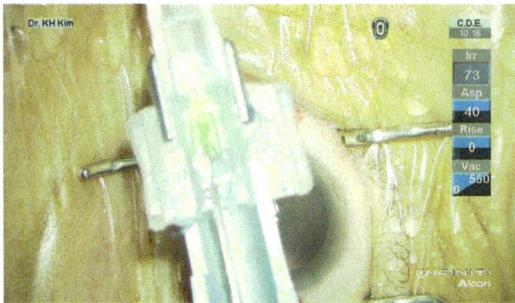
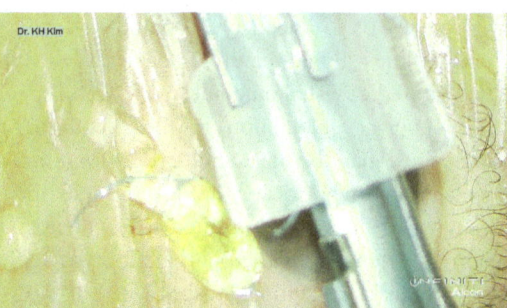
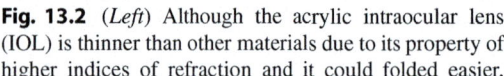

Fig. 13.2 (*Left*) Although the acrylic intraocular lens (IOL) is thinner than other materials due to its property of higher indices of refraction and it could folded easier,

(*Right*) IOLs with high diopter may be unsuitable for use with an injector for small incision, which could damage the IOL to be implanted

Implanting an IOL into an already crowded and small eye is technically challenging in eyes with microphthalmos. Furthermore, eyes with extreme hyperopia due to short axial length frequently require a higher diopter IOL than provided by manufacturers; therefore, these eyes may require more than one IOL. Additionally, the horizontal length of the capsular bag and the distance between ciliary sulci are often shorter than the total length of the IOL, hampering IOL implantation and proper positioning in the capsular bag or ciliary sulcus. Acrylic IOLs have higher indices of refraction than other materials, such as polymethyl methacrylate or silicone; therefore the thicknesses of these IOLs could be reduced more than those of IOLs made of other materials, making acrylic IOLs more useful for implantation into microphthalmic eyes. Although thinner than other IOLs, IOLs with high diopter may be unsuitable for use with an injector, because the IOL could not be folded and easily slid into the cartridge (Fig. 13.2). Manual insertion of the IOL using an IOL folding forceps and an IOL inserting forceps through a wider corneal incision may be advantageous for microphthalmic eyes requiring a higher diopter IOL. If an eye needs an IOL of higher diopter than manufactured, implantation of two or more IOLs, known as the piggyback technique [16, 22], can yield satisfactory outcomes. Emmetropia may be achieved by using two IOLs of equal power [23], or by using one IOL of the highest power available and the second IOL of the necessary supplementary power [15]. Although these IOLs can be

placed simultaneously into the capsular bag, the limited space in the capsular bag may make the implantation of more than one IOL technically challenging. Furthermore, opacification in the contact zone of the two IOLs, or interpseudophakic opacification, could occur postoperatively when two IOLs are placed in the capsular bag [3, 15, 24]. Cells proliferating at the IOL interface may displace the posteriorly located IOL more posteriorly. In addition, peripheral separation of the IOL optics and the resultant change in zonular tension may displace the entire capsular bag, resulting in a hyperopic shift. [24] Alternatively, the flatter central contact zone between IOLs due to capsular shrinkage may increase pressure on the IOL optic, with the central zone having less refractive power than the periphery and resulting in hyperopic shift. [25] Therefore, placing the higher power IOL into the capsular bag and the second IOL of less power into the ciliary sulcus is preferred to decrease interpseudophakic opacification and the resultant hyperopic shift (Fig. 13.3). Other advantages include a lower degree of spherical aberration and easier change in the IOL of supplementary power if needed in the future, although the risk of decentration is higher for the IOL located in the sulcus than in the capsular bag [15]. The scaffold for cellular ingrowth between the IOLs may be reduced by reducing the biocompatibility of the interface and increasing the physical distance between the IOL optics, placing an IOL made of silicone into the capsular bag and an acrylic IOL in the ciliary sulcus [26].

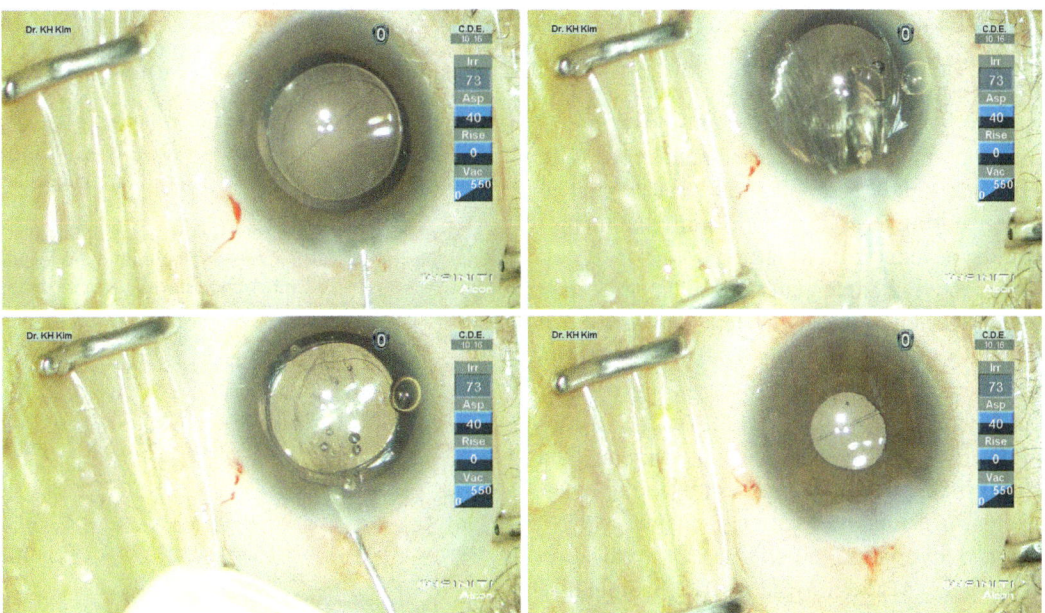

Fig. 13.3 Piggyback technique was used in a patient with high axial hyperopia. (*Top left*) The intraocular lens (IOL) of the highest power available was implanted in the capsular bag, and (*Top right*) the second IOL of the necessary supplementary power was implanted into the ciliary sulcus. (*Bottom Left and Right*) After checking the posi-

tion of IOLs, and injection of anticholinergics into the anterior chamber was done to secure IOLs in their position after the surgery. Residual refractive errors in this patient was measured as −0.25 diopter in a spherical equivalent 6 months postoperatively

Postoperative Considerations

The sclera in microphthalmic eyes is thickened and its permeability is reduced. This may lead to uveal effusions resulting from choroidal congestion secondary to impaired vortex venous drainage through the thick sclera and to resultant serous retinal detachment, which could be treated by vortex vein decompression or drainage of choroidal and/or subretinal fluid by air injection into the vitreous cavity [27]. Changes in transscleral hydrostatic pressure caused by postoperative hypotony may also induce uveal effusion. Therefore, postoperative intraocular pressure should be carefully evaluated and monitored. In addition, because inflammatory responses, which change osmotic gradients and vascular permeability, may be involved in the development or deterioration of uveal effusion, corticosteroids before and after surgery may prevent uveal effusion by minimizing intraocular

inflammation due to cataract surgery. However, no significant association was observed between steroid use and uveal effusion [6]. Additionally, preoperative medications to reduce intraocular pressure, such as acetazolamide and mannitol, may prevent uveal effusion by reducing fluctuations in intraocular pressure. However, the association between the use of acetazolamide or mannitol and the occurrence of uveal effusion has been found not to be significant [6], and treatment of these eyes with steroid, acetazolamide or mannitol did not significantly affect the occurrence of cystoid macular edema, which is highly prevalent in microphthalmic eyes after cataract surgery [6].

Eyes that develop visually significant interpseudophakic opacification after piggyback IOL implantation may be successfully treated by application of the neodymium-doped yttrium aluminum garnet (Nd: YAG) laser on the edge of the anterior capsulorhexis. This method is also successful in treating associated hyperopic shift, releasing tension on the lens complex, reducing hyperopia and unsealing the edge of the capsulorhexis from the lenses, providing a migration path for the lens epithelial cells [28]. Focusing tightly and using the least amount of energy during this procedure is important in preventing or reducing lens pitting.

Secondary angle closure glaucoma may occur if the ciliary body is rotated or pushed forward by uveal effusion [29]. Prophylactic peripheral iridotomy before or during cataract surgery may not significantly reduce the postoperative occurrence of angle closure glaucoma [6]. If malignant glaucoma occurs due to aqueous misdirection, medications, including cycloplegics, mydriatics and steroids, or application of the Nd: YAG laser to the anterior hyaloid face through an iridectomy could be attempted.

References

1. Duke-Elder S. Anomalies in the size of the eye. In: System of ophthalmology. St. Louis: Mosby; 1963. p. 488–95.
2. Auffarth GU, Blum M, Faller U, Tetz MR, Volcker HE. Relative anterior microphthalmos: morphometric analysis and its implications for cataract surgery. Ophthalmology. 2000;107:1555–60.
3. Wladis EJ, Gewirtz MB, Guo S. Cataract surgery in the small adult eye. Surv Ophthalmol. 2006;51:153–61.
4. Day AC, MacLaren RE, Bunce C, Stevens JD, Foster PJ. Outcomes of phacoemulsification and intraocular lens implantation in microphthalmos and nanophthalmos. J Cataract Refract Surg. 2013;39:87–96.
5. Carifi G, Safa F, Aiello F, Baumann C, Maurino V. Cataract surgery in small adult eyes. Br J Ophthalmol. 2014;98:1261–5.
6. Steijns D, Bijlsma WR, Van der Lelij A. Cataract surgery in patients with nanophthalmos. Ophthalmology. 2013;120:266–70.
7. Burgoyne C, Tello C, Katz LJ. Nanophthalmia and chronic angle-closure glaucoma. J Glaucoma. 2002;11:525–8.
8. Yalvac IS, Satana B, Ozkan G, Eksioglu U, Duman S. Management of glaucoma in patients with nanophthalmos. Eye (Lon Eng). 2008;22:838–43.
9. Singh OS, Simmons RJ, Brockhurst RJ, Trempe CL. Nanophthalmos: a perspective on identification and therapy. Ophthalmology. 1982;89:1006–12.
10. Seki M, Fukuchi T, Ueda J, et al. Nanophthalmos: quantitative analysis of anterior chamber angle configuration before and after cataract surgery. Br J Ophthalmol. 2012;96:1108–16.
11. Holladay JT, Gills JP, Leidlein J, Cherchio M. Achieving emmetropia in extremely short eyes with two piggyback posterior chamber intraocular lenses. Ophthalmology. 1996;103:1118–23.
12. Day AC, Foster PJ, Stevens JD. Accuracy of intraocular lens power calculations in eyes with axial length <22.00 mm. Clin Experiment Ophthalmol. 2012;40:855–62.
13. Aristodemou P, Knox Cartwright NE, Sparrow JM, Johnston RL. Formula choice: Hoffer Q, Holladay 1, or SRK/T and refractive outcomes in 8108 eyes after cataract surgery with biometry by partial coherence interferometry. J Cataract Refract Surg. 2011;37:63–71.
14. Jung KI, Yang JW, Lee YC, Kim SY. Cataract surgery in eyes with nanophthalmos and relative anterior microphthalmos. Am J Ophthalmol. 2012;153:1161–8. e1.
15. Baumeister M, Kohnen T. Scheimpflug measurement of intraocular lens position after piggyback implantation of foldable intraocular lenses in eyes with high hyperopia. J Cataract Refract Surg. 2006;32:2098–104.
16. Cao KY, Sit M, Braga-Mele R. Primary piggyback implantation of 3 intraocular lenses in nanophthalmos. J Cataract Refract Surg. 2007;33:727–30.
17. Yuzbasioglu E, Artunay O, Agachan A, Bilen H. Phacoemulsification in patients with nanophthalmos. Can J Ophthalmol J Canadien D'ophtalmologie. 2009;44:534–9.
18. Wu W, Dawson DG, Sugar A, et al. Cataract surgery in patients with nanophthalmos: results and complications. J Cataract Refract Surg. 2004;30:584–90.
19. Nihalani BR, Jani UD, Vasavada AR, Auffarth GU. Cataract surgery in relative anterior microphthalmos. Ophthalmology. 2005;112:1360–7.
20. Chalam KV, Gupta SK, Agarwal S, Shah VA. Sutureless limited vitrectomy for positive vitreous pressure in cataract surgery. Ophthalmic Surgery Lasers Imaging: Off J Int Soc Imaging Eye. 2005;36:518–22.
21. Arshinoff SA. Dispersive-cohesive viscoelastic soft shell technique. J Cataract Refract Surg. 1999;25:167–73.
22. Gayton JL, Sanders VN. Implanting two posterior chamber intraocular lenses in a case of microphthalmos. J Cataract Refract Surg. 1993;19:776–7.
23. Shugar JK, Lewis C, Lee A. Implantation of multiple foldable acrylic posterior chamber lenses in the capsular bag for high hyperopia. J Cataract Refract Surg. 1996;22 Suppl 2:1368–72.
24. Shugar JK, Schwartz T. Interpseudophakos Elschnig pearls associated with late hyperopic shift: a complication of piggyback posterior chamber intraocular

lens implantation. J Cataract Refract Surg. 1999;25:863–7.

25. Findl O, Menapace R, Georgopoulos M, Kiss B, Petternel V, Rainer G. Morphological appearance and size of contact zones of piggyback intraocular lenses. J Cataract Refract Surg. 2001;27:219–23.

26. Shugar JK, Keeler S. Interpseudophakos intraocular lens surface opacification as a late complication of piggyback acrylic posterior chamber lens implantation. J Cataract Refract Surg. 2000;26:448–55.

27. Brockhurst RJ. Vortex vein decompression for nanophthalmic uveal effusion. Arch Ophthalmol (Chicago, Ill: 1960). 1980;98:1987–90.

28. Gayton JL, Van der Karr M, Sanders V. Neodymium:YAG treatment of interlenticular opacification in a secondary piggyback case. J Cataract Refract Surg. 2001;27:1511–3.

29. Kimbrough RL, Trempe CS, Brockhurst RJ, Simmons RJ. Angle-closure glaucoma in nanophthalmos. Am J Ophthalmol. 1979;88:572–9.

Cataract Surgery in Vitrectomized Eyes

14

Cataract formation is the most common complication of pars plana vitrectomy (PPV), with the incidence of new or progressive lens opacity after vitrectomy being as high as 80 % within 2 years [1, 2]. Patients with cataract after PPV are at a high risk of intraoperative and postoperative complications due to anatomical differences between the vitrectomized and unoperated ones. Several factors must be considered before, during and after surgery to achieve successful outcomes in these patients.

Preoperative Considerations

Because vitrectomized eyes could potentially experience sequelae of the original retinal disease and retinal surgery, the benefits and risks of cataract surgery must be carefully evaluated. In addition to reviewing medical records, the potential acuity meter is useful and more accurate than the pinhole test in predicting visual acuity after cataract surgery [3]. Use of illuminated near card assessment during preoperative evaluation has shown greater accuracy than potential acuity meter measurements, although the former shows a tendency toward overestimation [4]. Careful and thorough evaluations of ocular structures and sequelae are of utmost importance in preparing for intraoperative challenges and designing a rigorous surgical strategy. Compromised ocular structures and sequelae after PPV include conjunctival or episcleral scarring, unhealthy corneal endothelial cells, zonular weakness, emulsified silicone oil in the anterior chamber, poor dilation of the pupil, new vessels of the iris and retinal problems such as macular edema and retinal break. Patients undergone PPV should be properly counseled and informed consent should be obtained. In particular, patients should be informed that secondary interventions may be required to address postoperative complications such as retinal detachment and corneal decompensation, and, where necessary, patients should be informed that postoperative visual outcomes may be affected by retinal health and sequelae after previous PPV.

Despite developments in the technology of biometry, accurate measurements of axial length remain challenging, because the normal anatomy is altered in vitrectomized eyes. Furthermore, because a high percentage of vitrectomized eyes have high myopia, optical biometry using partial coherence laser interferometry could yield more accurate and reproducible results [5], by avoiding corneal indentations made by the ultrasound probe, improving patient fixation on the measuring beam and preventing eccentric measurement on the staphyloma. However, although myopic shift, which occurs when using applanation A-scan ultrasound in cataract patients with PPV [6], was not observed, the results of optical biometry were not as accurate in vitrectomized as in nonvitrectomized eyes [7]. Optical biometry measures axial length from the corneal surface to the retinal pigment

© Springer-Verlag Berlin Heidelberg 2016
W.S. Kim, K.H. Kim, *Challenges in Cataract Surgery*, DOI 10.1007/978-3-662-46092-4_14

epithelium, whereas ultrasound biometry measures axial length in reference to the internal limiting membrane [8]. In addition, anatomical alterations differ in various retinal diseases. Thus, the accuracy of axial length measurements will depend on both the disease and the method of measurement. If the validity of biometric measurement is suspect, both ultrasound and optical biometry should be performed [9]. Accurate measurement of axial length may also be affected by the silicone oil often used to fill vitrectomized eyes during PPV. The speed of ultrasound waves is slower in silicone oil than in vitreous humor [10], and multiple fluid interfaces and poor penetration due to sound absorption by oil can result in measurement errors. Thus, axial length in silicone oil filled eyes will be overestimated using A-scan ultrasound [11]. Accurate axial length can therefore be calculated by multiplying the measured axial length by a conversion factor of 0.71 for silicone oil with a viscosity of 1300 centistokes [11]. Because higher viscosity results in greater changes in refraction and axial length [12], other conversion factors must be for silicone oil of viscosity other than 1300 centistokes. As light is less affected than sound waves by passage through different media, the correction factor for axial length calculations is much smaller for infrared light than for ultrasound. Thus, axial length measurements in pseudophakic and silicone oil-filled eyes are more accurate when determined by infrared [7]. If transmission of laser light into the retina is possible (e.g., in a silicone filled eye with less dense cataract, no corneal opacity and good patient fixation), optical biometry using partial coherence interferometry is preferred, as it is more accurate in predicting postoperative refractive error than A-scan ultrasound biometry using an immersion technique in silicone oil-filled eye [13]. An encircling procedure, which is often performed alone or with PPV for retinal detachment, alters the shape and axial length of the eyeball, causing visually significant refractive error. Axial eye length is also significantly increased by surgery (median 0.77 mm 1 month after surgery), although this elongation was reduced by 0.20 mm 1 year postoperatively [14]. Therefore, patients who may undergo encircling band removal should be warned that there is a risk of hyperopic shift, albeit low.

Several factors should be considered when selecting IOLs in patients with a history of previous PPV. IOLs made of silicone must be avoided, as vitrectomized eyes may undergo additional PPV with silicone oil tamponade. Silicone oil used during PPV may adhere to the IOL surface and manifest as a thick coating with droplet formation on the lens surface; this coating cannot be easily removed by an instrument or irrigation during PPV [15]. Furthermore, exposure of a silicone IOL to a silicone oil could lead to opacification or discoloration of the IOL during the late postoperative period [16]. Other IOL materials such as acrylate and polymethyl methacrylate are preferred because they interact less with silicone oil and adherent oil can be easily removed during surgery [17]. IOLs with a large sized optic and squared edges, which may provide a better view during fundus examination, may be advantageous for following-up the results of the original retinal pathology after cataract surgery. Yellow-colored blue light-filter IOLs, which were designed to reduce the absorption of ultraviolet (UV) and short-wavelength visible light, may reduce ocular damage and the progression of age related macular degeneration. A randomized clinical trial showed that yellow colored IOLs had no intraoperative or functional disadvantages compared with clear UV-filter IOLs [18]. Therefore, yellow-tinted IOLs may be useful for vitrectomized eyes, which have underlying vitreoretinal pathology, as well as possibly providing macular protection. Multifocal IOLs, which have two or more focal points, extending their range of vision but with reduced contrast sensitivity and photic phenomena, are not an ideal option for eyes with a history of PPV, as their contrast sensitivity is often already affected by the underlying vitreoretinal pathology. Furthermore, impaired visual outcome could impede the physician's view, preventing thorough follow-up fundus examinations and compromising surgical view during additional PPV.

Intraoperative Considerations

Conjunctival and episcleral scarring after PPV may limit the creation of a scleral tunnel incision due to severe synechia and vascularization. Therefore, clear corneal incisions are preferred in vitrectomized eyes, even if incisions are larger than 2.2 mm. If scleral rigidity is low and the risk of hypotony during surgery is increased, a 23 or 25 gauge infusion cannula can be inserted at pars plana transconjunctivally to maintain proper intraocular pressure and prevent associated complications. Cannula insertion may also provide additional capsular support in post-PPV eyes that lack vitreous support to float the lens (Fig. 14.1).

Inadequate preoperative mydriasis and fluctuation in pupil size during surgery may occur in cataract patients with a history of vitrectomy [19]. Synechiolysis and pupil dilating maneuvers, including intracameral mydriatics, pupillary membrane dissection and expanding the pupil using ophthalmic viscosurgical devices (OVD) or iris hooks (see Chap. 4), can be utilized to gain adequate access to the lens at the start of phacoemulsification. Fluctuation of pupil size in vitrectomized eyes may be associated with zonular laxity as well as absence of vitreous support. Deepening of the anterior chamber is frequently observed in vitrectomized eyes and is often associated with pupil dilation and a concave iris configuration (Fig. 14.2). This phenomenon, called lens-iris diaphragm retropulsion syndrome (LIDRS), is more frequent in eyes with extensive or multiple vitrectomy than in eyes with a lesser degree of vitrectomy because this syndrome is caused predominantly by loosened zonular suspension [20]. Weakened zonules and lack of a vitreous body could enable fluids to move gradually through the enlarged intervals of the zonules, increasing the volume of the vitreous cavity and the pressure of the posterior compartment. This may result in the anterior excursion of the iris-diaphragm, presenting as initial deepening and sudden shallowing or collapse of the anterior

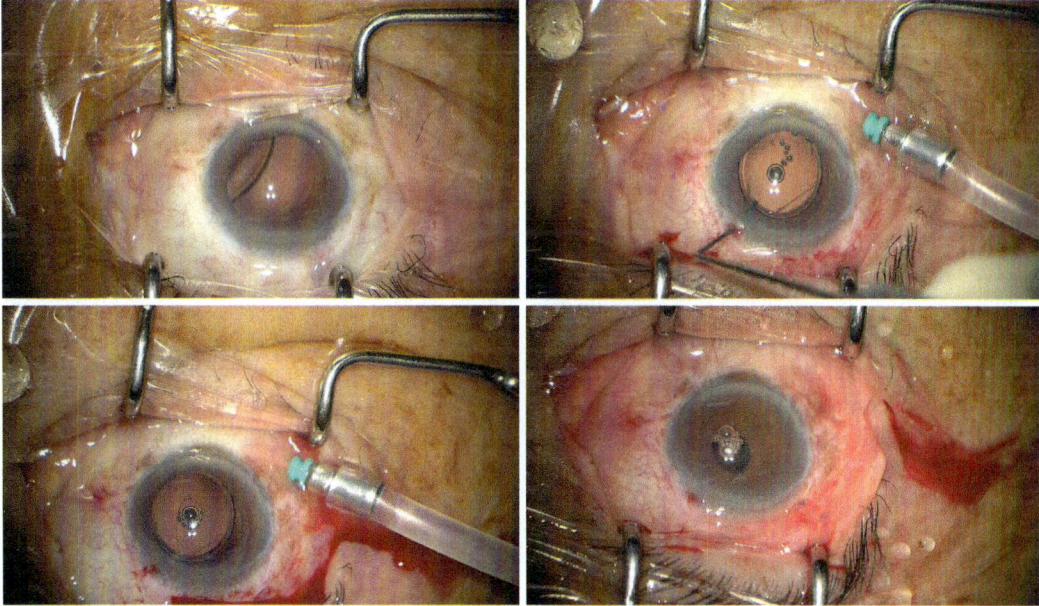

Fig. 14.1 (*Top Left*) For eyes after pars plana vitrectomy (PPV), (*Top Right*) an infusion cannula inserted at pars plana could be employed during surgeries for the anterior segment. In addition to aid in maintaining intraocular pressure stable during intraocular manipulation, (*Bottom Left*) an infusion flow from the posterior segment could take the place of vitreous support to float the intraocular lens (IOL), and this could be employed to provide additional capsular support during cataract surgery in post-PPV eyes. (*Bottom Right*) The scleral fixation of the dislocated IOL was performed safely and successfully in this patient, who was referred to my clinic due to the IOL dislocation after total vitrectomy and intrascleral tunnel fixation of the IOL

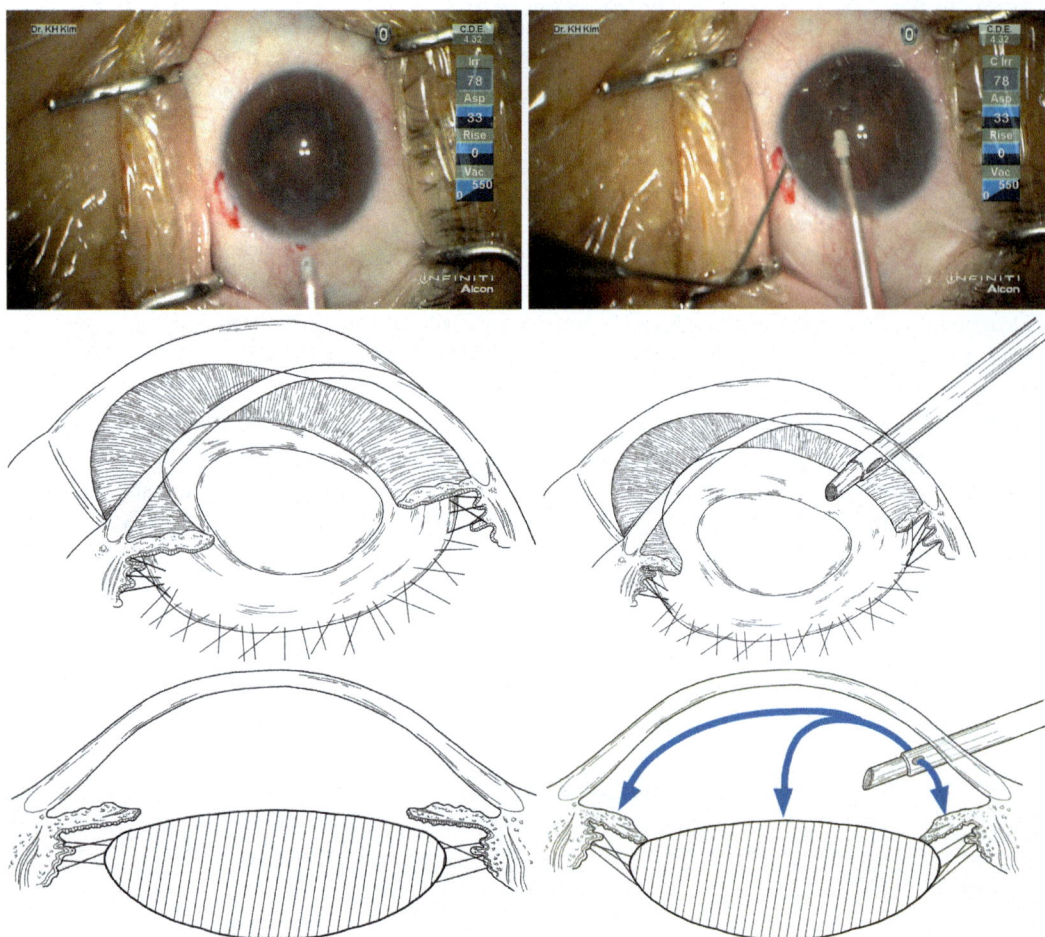

Fig. 14.2 (*Left Column*) In eyes with thinly stretched zonules and underdeveloped ciliary bodies, (*Right Column*) an infusion into the anterior chamber may deepen the anterior chamber and push iris posteriorly, causing marked pupillary dilation and patient's discom-fort. This phenomenon, called lens-iris diaphragm retropulsion syndrome, is more frequent in eyes with extensive or multiple vitrectomy than in eyes with a lesser degree of vitrectomy because loosened zonular suspension is considered as its predominant cause

chamber as well as pupillary miosis (infusion deviation syndrome) [21]. Therefore, reducing bottle height and proportionately reducing the vacuum and flow rate during phacoemulsification can prevent further complications. Meticulous manipulation of a foot pedal to slowly increase infusion pressure while inserting hand-pieces for phacoemulsification can help stabilize the anterior chamber. If LIDRS occurs despite these techniques, a second instrument can be used to immediately lift the iris margins, equalizing the pressure between the anterior and posterior chambers, relieving patient discomfort and reversing LIDRS (Fig. 14.3) [22]. In addition, if the anterior chamber suddenly becomes shallow,

increasing infusion pressure by raising the bottle height should be avoided, because this may exacerbate shallowing of the anterior chamber and lead to total collapse. An overly shallow or collapsed chamber can be expanded by injecting an OVD and performing phacoemulsification in the anterior chamber, which keeps the irrigation tip anterior to the iris plane. Deepening of the anterior chamber in vitrectomized eyes reduces accessibility of instruments and hand pieces of phacoemulsification and irrigation-aspiration of the lens. Therefore, they should be inserted more deeply and more perpendicular to the iris plane than in uncomplicated cataract surgery. Despite limited manipulation ability, significant care

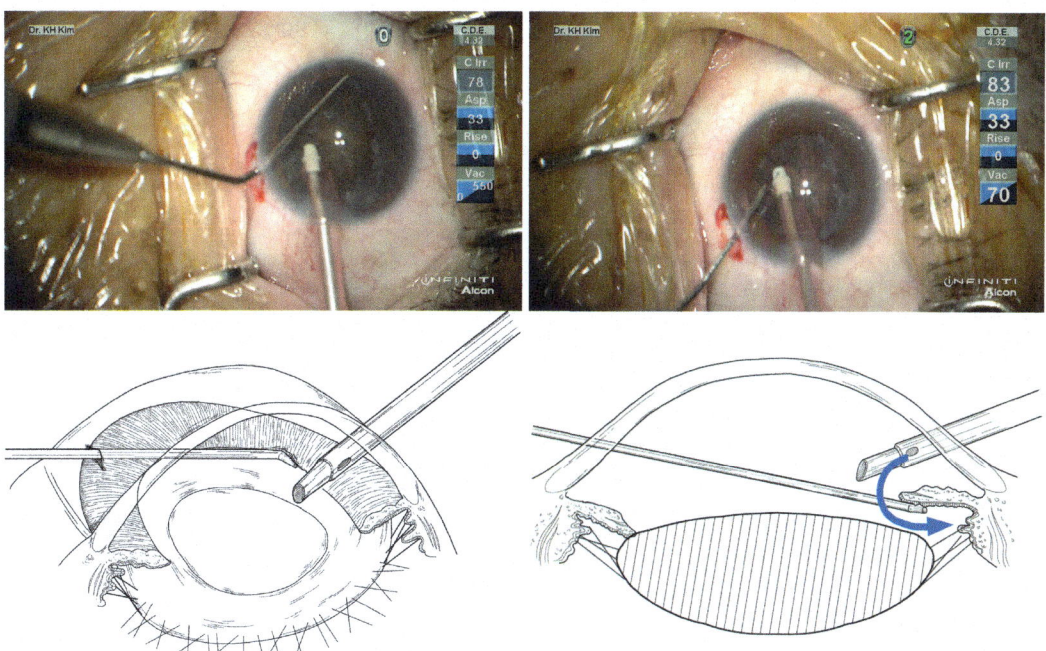

Fig. 14.3 (*Top Left and Right*) Lens-iris diaphragm retropulsion syndrome (LIDRS), characterized by the marked dilatation of the pupil and concave configuration of the iris, could be reversed by a second instrument. (*Bottom Left and Right*) An instrument such as chopper or spatula can be used to immediately lift the iris margins for the irrigation flow to be entered into the posterior chamber between the iris and lens capsule. Thus, this maneuver could equalize the pressure between the anterior and posterior chambers, relieving patient discomfort and reversing LIDRS

should be taken not to induce further damage to the weakened zonules (Fig. 14.4). Because post-PPV eyes may experience pain and discomfort due to the pupil dilating maneuver and LIDRS, peribulbar/retrobulbar anesthesia or intracameral administration of preservative-free lidocaine hydrochloride 1 % may be preferred to make patients more comfortable during surgery.

Anterior subcapsular tissue plaque, which may develop after exposure to silicone oil [23], may prevent complete continuous curvilinear capsulorhexis (CCC). Intraocular scissors or Vannas scissors may be helpful in completing CCC by cutting the fibrotic subcapsular tissue in the direction of the CCC. Although vitrectomized eyes are not at a higher risk of anterior capsular opening contraction [24], a larger sized CCC would be more beneficial. Preexisting zonular weakness may be further compromised by capsular fibrosis and shrinkage postoperatively, increasing the risk of postoperative complications such as IOL dislocation. Furthermore, vit-

rectomized eyes generally require continuous follow up by fundoscopic examination due to the original retinal disease that led to the vitrectomy. However, areas of anterior capsular fibrosis may interfere with the examiner's view, especially during examination of the peripheral retina.

Posterior capsular opacity or plaque is the most common intraoperative problem in eyes that have undergone previous vitrectomy [21, 25–27]. Centrally located opacity or plaque has a significant effect on visual outcomes and should therefore be removed completely by using capsular forceps to peel off the plaque, starting from its edge, or by using a capsule polisher to polish off the plaque. Because the posterior capsule is flaccid and mobile in post-PPV eyes [19, 27], meticulous manipulation of instruments is important so as not to disrupt the posterior capsule during this procedure and during removal of the cortical material. If the opacity or plaque is quite dense, it can be removed by primary posterior CCC during surgery or postoperatively by posterior capsulotomy using

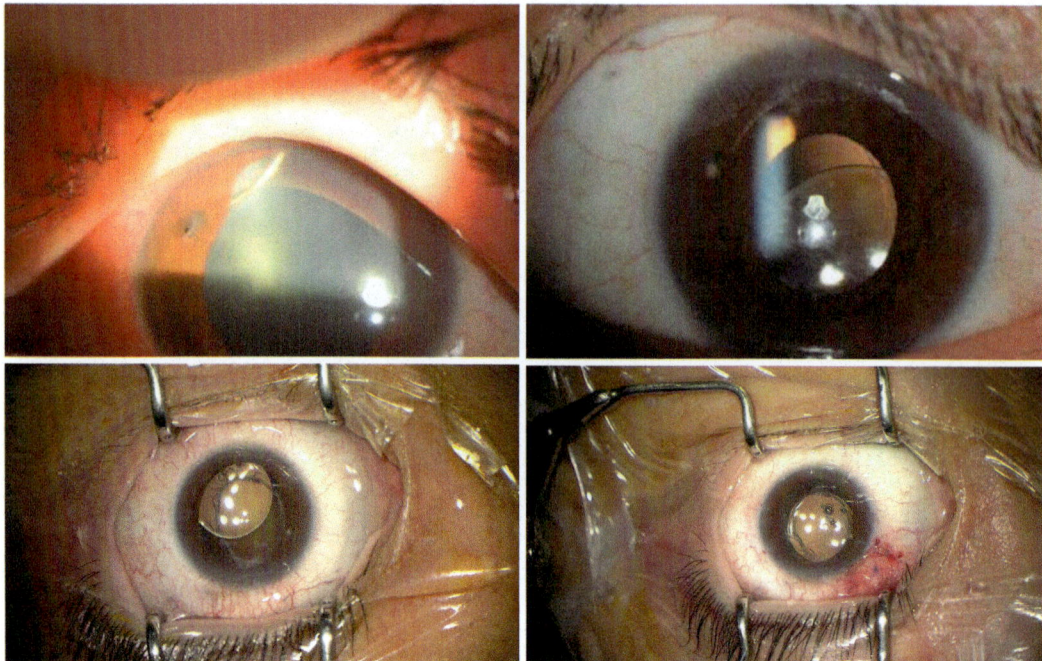

Fig. 14.4 A 31-year-old man with a symptom of visual discomfort and progressively decreased vision for 2 months was referred to anterior segment service by the retinal surgeon. (*Top Left*) His medical record revealed total vitrectomy and cataract surgery due to penetrating trauma 3 months prior. (*Top Right*) Slitlamp examination revealed the intraocular lens (IOL) positioned in the sulcus and dislocated inferiorly. This complication was possibly caused by the extensive vitrectomy on the vitreous base, as described by the retinal surgeon on the medical record, and resultant weakness of the zonular structure. This case shows that significant care should be taken not to induce further damage to the already weakened zonules during cataract surgery in eyes with a history of vitrectomy. (*Bottom Left and Right*) Inferiorly dislocated IOL in this patient was successfully repositioned using scleral fixation technique

a neodymium-doped yttrium aluminum garnet (Nd: YAG) laser (the author's preference).

Postoperative Considerations

The most frequent postoperative complication in post-PPV eyes is posterior capsular opacity (PCO), with an incidence of 31.8–51 % after a mean 19 months [25, 27]. This incidence is much higher than in patients after uncomplicated cataract surgery (11.8 % at 12 months and 20.7 % at 36 months) [28]. Furthermore, this incidence has been reported to be 58 % and 100 % when expandable gas and silicone oil, respectively, were used at vitrectomy [27]. As in patients with uncomplicated cataract, this complication in post-PPV eyes can usually be successfully managed by posterior capsulotomy using an Nd: YAG laser. Alternatively, this complication may be reduced by complete removal of lens epithelial cells with gentle and meticulous capsular polishing, although this is often difficult in vitrectomized eyes due to the flaccid and mobile nature of the posterior capsule.

A compromised zonular structure, which occurs frequently in vitrectomized eyes [21, 25, 27], may lead to late in-the-bag dislocation of the IOL. Indeed, a history of vitrectomy was reported to be the second most frequent condition observed in eyes with in-the-bag dislocation of the IOL [29]. Although endocapsular devices such as capsular tension rings (CTRs) can be implanted to stabilize capsular bags in patients with nonprogressive zonulopathy, zonular weakness in post-PPV eyes may be progressive and lead to in-the-bag CTR and IOL dislocation [30]. Iris or scleral fixation techniques for repositioning of

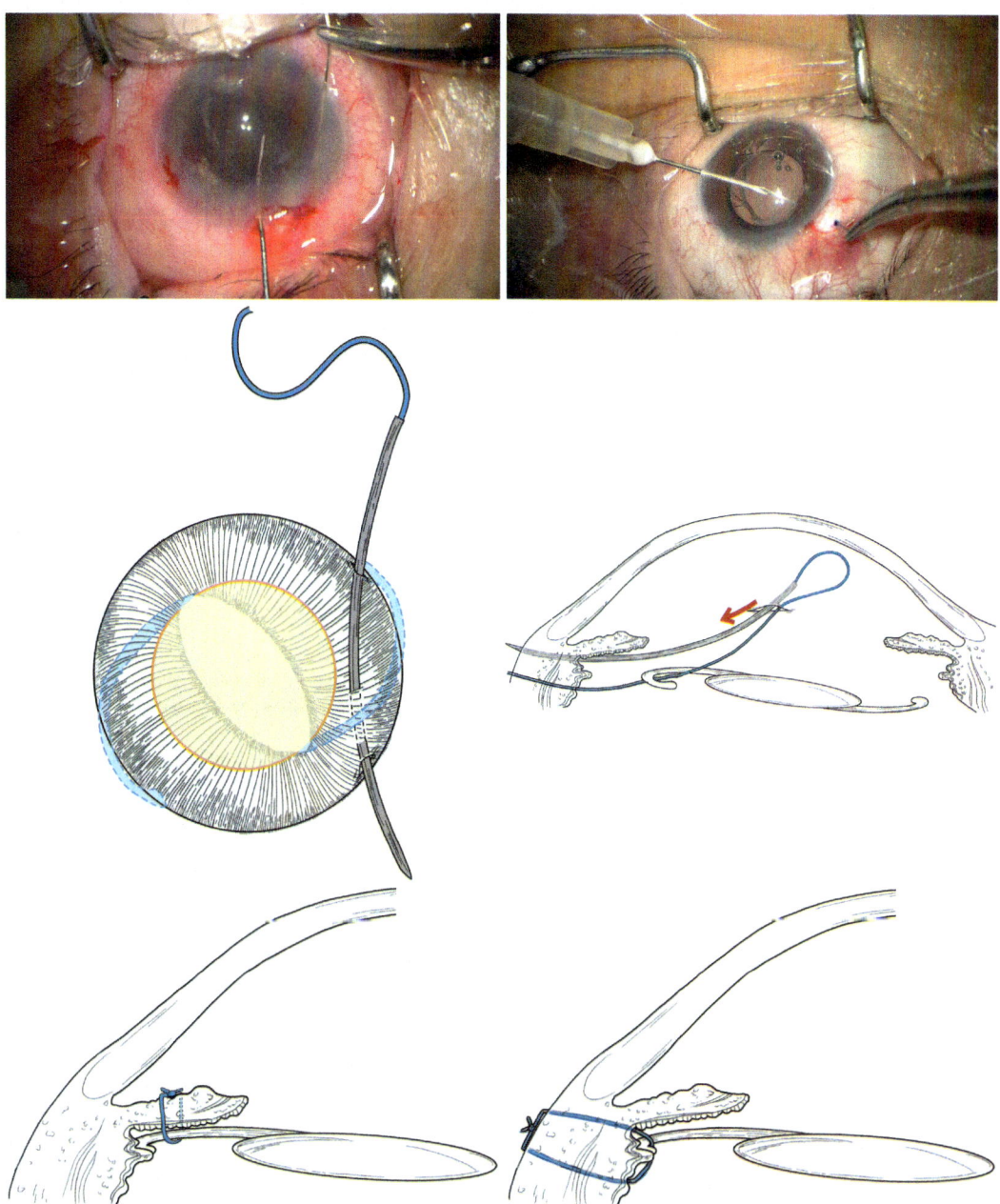

Fig. 14.5 Intraocular lens (IOL) dislocation is frequent complication of cataract surgery in vitrectomized eyes, which may be caused by a compromised zonular structure. This complication could be treated successfully using the iris fixation (*Left Column*) or scleral fixation (*Right Column*) techniques. Iris fixation and scleral fixation techniques are known to have similar efficacy in the repositioning of dislocated intraocular lenses. It is also known that the iris fixation had several disadvantages, including induced astigmatism, immediate postoperative inflammation, earlier recurrence, and less stable refraction compared to the scleral fixation technique, although operation time was shorter for the iris fixation

dislocated IOLs can correct this complication effectively and safely, although use of these techniques should be decided after considering their advantages and disadvantages in individual patients (Fig. 14.5) [31]. The additional cost of the device and the relatively low incidence of

IOL dislocation after cataract surgery (0.2–3 %) suggest that routine prophylactic implantation of endocapsular devices in post-PPV eyes is not appropriate.

The retinal pathology that led to vitrectomy may have an impact on final visual outcomes. For example, Snellen visual acuity was found to improve in 84.6 % of eyes previously treated for macular hole, in 85.7 % of eyes treated for 'macula-on' retinal detachment, in 66.7 % of eyes treated for 'macula-off' retinal detachment, and in 57.1 % of eyes treated for diabetic retinopathy [21]. However, to maximize visual outcomes after cataract surgery in vitrectomized eyes, patients should be followed-up periodically for progression or development of retinal comorbidities and treated prophylactically, including with topical NSAIDs, to prevent the development of macular edema.

References

1. Cherfan GM, Michels RG, de Bustros S, Enger C, Glaser BM. Nuclear sclerotic cataract after vitrectomy for idiopathic epiretinal membranes causing macular pucker. Am J Ophthalmol. 1991;111: 434–8.
2. Hsuan JD, Brown NA, Bron AJ, Patel CK, Rosen PH. Posterior subcapsular and nuclear cataract after vitrectomy. J Cataract Refract Surg. 2001;27:437–44.
3. Uy HS, Munoz VM. Comparison of the potential acuity meter and pinhole tests in predicting postoperative visual acuity after cataract surgery. J Cataract Refract Surg. 2005;31:548–52.
4. Chang MA, Airiani S, Miele D, Braunstein RE. A comparison of the potential acuity meter (PAM) and the illuminated near card (INC) in patients undergoing phacoemulsification. Eye (Lond). 2006;20: 1345–51.
5. Findl O, Drexler W, Menapace R, Heinzl H, Hitzenberger CK, Fercher AF. Improved prediction of intraocular lens power using partial coherence interferometry. J Cataract Refract Surg. 2001;27:861–7.
6. Patel D, Rahman R, Kumarasamy M. Accuracy of intraocular lens power estimation in eyes having phacovitrectomy for macular holes. J Cataract Refract Surg. 2007;33:1760–2.
7. Manvikar SR, Allen D, Steel DH. Optical biometry in combined phacovitrectomy. J Cataract Refract Surg. 2009;35:64–9.
8. Hitzenberger CK, Drexler W, Dolezal C, et al. Measurement of the axial length of cataract eyes by laser Doppler interferometry. Invest Ophthalmol Vis Sci. 1993;34:1886–93.
9. Shousha MA, Yoo SH. Cataract surgery after pars plana vitrectomy. Curr Opin Ophthalmol. 2010;21:45–9.
10. Hoffer KJ. Ultrasound velocities for axial eye length measurement. J Cataract Refract Surg. 1994;20:554–62.
11. Murray DC, Potamitis T, Good P, Kirkby GR, Benson MT. Biometry of the silicone oil-filled eye. Eye (Lond). 1999;13(Pt 3a):319–24.
12. Seo MS, Lim ST, Kim HD, Park BI. Changes in refraction and axial length according to the viscosity of intraocular silicone oil. Korean J Ophthalmol KJO. 1999;13:25–9.
13. Kunavisarut P, Poopattanakul P, Intarated C, Pathanapitoon K. Accuracy and reliability of IOL master and A-scan immersion biometry in silicone oil-filled eyes. Eye (Lond). 2012;26:1344–8.
14. Malukiewicz-Wisniewska G, Stafiej J. Changes in axial length after retinal detachment surgery. Eur J Ophthalmol. 1999;9:115–9.
15. Apple DJ, Federman JL, Krolicki TJ, et al. Irreversible silicone oil adhesion to silicone intraocular lenses. A clinicopathologic analysis. Ophthalmology. 1996;103:1555–61; discussion 1561–2.
16. Werner L. Causes of intraocular lens opacification or discoloration. J Cataract Refract Surg. 2007;33:713–26.
17. Khawly JA, Lambert RJ, Jaffe GJ. Intraocular lens changes after short- and long-term exposure to intraocular silicone oil. An in vivo study. Ophthalmology. 1998;105:1227–33.
18. Falkner-Radler CI, Benesch T, Binder S. Blue light-filter intraocular lenses in vitrectomy combined with cataract surgery: results of a randomized controlled clinical trial. Am J Ophthalmol. 2008;145:499–503.
19. McDermott ML, Puklin JE, Abrams GW, Eliott D. Phacoemulsification for cataract following pars plana vitrectomy. Ophthalmic Surg Lasers. 1997;28:558–64.
20. Ghosh S, Best K, Steel DH. Lens-iris diaphragm retropulsion syndrome during phacoemulsification in vitrectomized eyes. J Cataract Refract Surg. 2013;39:1852–8.
21. Ahfat FG, Yuen CH, Groenewald CP. Phacoemulsification and intraocular lens implantation following pars plana vitrectomy: a prospective study. Eye (Lond). 2003;17:16–20.
22. Cheung CM, Hero M. Stabilization of anterior chamber depth during phacoemulsification cataract surgery in vitrectomized eyes. J Cataract Refract Surg. 2005;31:2055–7.
23. Koch FH, Cusumano A, Seifert P, Mougharbel M, Augustin AJ. Ultrastructure of the anterior lens capsule after vitrectomy with silicone oil injection. Correlation of clinical and morphological features. Documenta Ophthalmologica Adv Ophthalmol. 1995;91:233–42.

24. Matsuda H, Kato S, Hayashi Y, et al. Anterior capsular contraction after cataract surgery in vitrectomized eyes. Am J Ophthalmol. 2001;132:108–9.

25. Grusha YO, Masket S, Miller KM. Phacoemulsification and lens implantation after pars plana vitrectomy. Ophthalmology. 1998;105:287–94.

26. Chang MA, Parides MK, Chang S, Braunstein RE. Outcome of phacoemulsification after pars plana vitrectomy. Ophthalmology. 2002;109:948–54.

27. Pinter SM, Sugar A. Phacoemulsification in eyes with past pars plana vitrectomy: case–control study. J Cataract Refract Surg. 1999;25:556–61.

28. Schaumberg DA, Dana MR, Christen WG, Glynn RJ. A systematic overview of the incidence of posterior capsule opacification. Ophthalmology. 1998;105:1213–21.

29. Davis D, Brubaker J, Espandar L, et al. Late in-the-bag spontaneous intraocular lens dislocation: evaluation of 86 consecutive cases. Ophthalmology. 2009;116:664–70.

30. Werner L, Zaugg B, Neuhann T, Burrow M, Tetz M. In-the-bag capsular tension ring and intraocular lens subluxation or dislocation: a series of 23 cases. Ophthalmology. 2012;119:266–71.

31. Kim KH, Kim WS. Comparison of clinical outcomes of iris fixation and scleral fixation as treatment for intraocular lens dislocation. Am J Ophthalmol. 2015;160:463–469.e1.

As recent progress in cataract surgery including anesthesia, small incision surgery, introduction of various medications allow us to perform cataract surgery with least complication. However, in addition to many bleeding disorders from vascular fragility, thrombocytopenia, defective platelet function, abnormalities in clotting factors, disseminated intravascular coagulation (DIC), and related systemic disorders (renal, hepatic, and rheumatologic disorders), ingestion of many drugs alter normal hemostasis, make cataract surgery more challenging.

Red Cell Diseases

Iron deficiency anemia, Anemia of chronic disease, Alpha and Beta thalassemia, Sideroblastic anemia, Vitamin B6 deficiency, Vitamin B 12 deficiency, myelodysplastic disorders, Polychromasia, Autoimmune ant intravascular hemolytic anemias, Sickle cell disease, Aplastic anemia etc.

White Blood Cell Disorders

Leukopenia (Neutropenia, Deficiencies of other circulating phagocytes, Lymphocytopenia), Leukocytosis and Leukemoid reactions, Neutrophilia etc.

Hemostasis Disorders

Table 15.1

Preoperative Considerations

As with other surgical procedures, histories about bleeding tendencies in the past should be included in questioinaires before the operation, known hereditary conditions causing bleeding, acquired systemic ailment disturbing normal clotting. A lot of dietary supplement should be inspected for their impact on normal clotting phenomenon. (e.g., Herb, Coenzyme Q1, Omega-3 fish oil, Vitamins etc.) [1, 2].

Patients should asked to stop using medication before the day of the operation. Although current surgical technique allows us to complete cataract surgery without bleeding, these patients with risk of bleeding tendency should be informed about possible bleeding accidents that might occur during the cataract surgery, especially when more complicated surgical procedure is anticipated (Table 15.2).

As there are a lot of patients who under medications such as antiplatelet and anticoagulant medication as there are increase in cardiac interventions with increasing life expectancy, they need to get special attentions before the surgery [3–5].

© Springer-Verlag Berlin Heidelberg 2016
W.S. Kim, K.H. Kim, *Challenges in Cataract Surgery*, DOI 10.1007/978-3-662-46092-4_15

Table 15.1 Characteristic patterns of bleeding in systemic disorders of hemostatsis

Type of disorder	Sites of bleeding	Examples
Platelet-vascular disorders	Superficial surfaces; Petechiae, ecchymoses Common: oral, nasal, gastrointestinal, genitourinary	Thrombocytopenia, functional platelet disorder, vascular fragility, disseminated intravascular coagulation, liver disease
Coagulation factor deficiency	Deep tissues; Hematomas Common: joint, muscle, retroperitoneal	Inherited coagulation factor deficiency, acquired inhibitor, anticoagulation, disseminated intravascular coagulation, liver disease

Reference: Goldman-Cecil Medicine, 171, 1154–1159.e2, Table 171–1

Table 15.2 Screening assays for hemostasis

Laboratory test	Aspect of hemostasis tested	Causes of abnormalities
Blood counts and peripheral blood smear	Platelet count and morphologic features	Thrombocytopenia, thrombocytosis, gray platelet and giant platelet syndromes
Prothrombin time	Factor VII dependent pathways	Vitamin K deficiency and warfarin, liver disease, DIC, factor deficiency (VII, V, X, II), factor inhibitor
Partial thromboplastin time	Factor XI, IX, and VIII dependent pathways	Heparin, DIC, lupus anticoagulant, factor deficiency (XI, IX, VIII, V, X, II), factor inhibitor
Thrombin time	Fibrinogen	Heparin, hypofibrinogenemia, dysfibrinogenemia, DIC
Platelet function analysis	Platelet and Von Willebrand factor function	Aspirin, Von Willebrand disease, storage pool disease

Reference: Andreoli and Carpenter's Cecil Essentials of Medicine, 51, 544–563, table 51-1

Intraoperative Considerations

I advise to performed surgery under low vacuum to minimize iris damage which might be the major cause for bleeding during cataract surgery. If there's large capsular tear and zonular compromise, and does not allow in the bag and sulcus placement of IOL, alternative options for IOL placement (such as sclera fixation of IOL and Iris fixation or IOL) might cause serious bleeding. Further progress to IOL placement should be a concern in patient with bleeding tendencies, and should be considered and should be discussed with the patients before the surgery.

References

1. Ansell J. Effects of dietary supplements on hemostasis. Thromb Res. 2005;117:45–7.
2. Basila D, Yuan CS. Effects of dietary supplements on coagulation and platelet function. Thromb Res. 2005;117:49–53.
3. Kara-Junior N, Santhiago MR, Almeida HG, Raiza AC. Safety of warfarin therapy during cataract surgery under topical anesthesia. Arq Bras Oftalmol. 2015;78:173–4.
4. Jamula E, Anderson J, Douketis JD. Safety of continuing warfarin therapy during cataract surgery: a systematic review and meta-analysis. Thromb Res. 2009;124:292–9.
5. Kadyan A, Edmunds MR. Intraocular surgery with warfarin anticoagulation. J Cataract Refract Surg. 2010;36:701–2.

Cataract Surgery in Patients with Corneal Diseases

Corneal diseases may limit surgical techniques during cataract surgery and may lead to undesirable surgical results. Furthermore, cataract surgery may contribute to the progression of preexisting corneal diseases [1]. Preoperative identification of corneal morbidity and appropriate perioperative management, including relevant surgical techniques, are essential for surgery to have optimal outcomes.

Corneal Epithelial Disease

Preoperative Considerations

Because the anterior corneal surface, including the tear film, is responsible for most of the refractive power of the eye, a healthy ocular surface and tear film are crucial for good visual outcomes after cataract surgery [2]. Although dry eye disease in cataract patients can be exacerbated postoperatively and may be associated with unpleasant situations perioperatively [3], more severe ocular surface diseases, such as graft-versus-host disease, ocular cicatricial pemphigoid and Stevens-Johnson syndrome, could result in serious postoperative complications such as corneal melting or reactivation of the disease [4–6]. Surgery should be postponed in these patients until the inflammatory component is fully controlled and disease activity is markedly reduced. In patients with chronic graft-versus-host disease, aggressive lubrication is sufficient for surgery [5], whereas, in patients with other diseases, preoperative systemic immunosuppressive therapy may be necessary to reduce inflammation.

Ocular surface diseases in cataract patients may also give rise to inaccurate biometric measurements. Ocular surface abnormalities may interfere with accurate keratometry measurements, resulting in postoperative ametropia and patient dissatisfaction due to errors in intraocular lens power calculations. The risk of errors may be reduced by using more than one method of obtaining keratometric readings and comparing their consistency. Measurements before the instillation of eye drops or applanation tonometry may also result in more accurate biometric readings [2].

Intraoperative Considerations

The choice of wound location should depend on the disease entity. For example, scleral tunnel incisions may be more suitable than corneal incisions in patients with Mooren's ulcer, thus minimizing the risks of postoperative corneal melting [6]. In contrast, clear corneal incisions may be more appropriate in patients with diseases such as rheumatoid arthritis and Stevens-Johnson syndrome because any insult to the sclera in patients with these diseases could trigger inflammatory cascades and exacerbate disease progression [6, 7].

W.S. Kim, K.H. Kim, *Challenges in Cataract Surgery*, DOI 10.1007/978-3-662-46092-4_16

Abnormalities in the ocular surface may not only have a negative effect on visual outcomes, but impede surgical views during cataract extraction. Intraoperative views may be improved in patients with evaporative dry eye by the application of hydroxyl methylcellulose 2 % gel, as this gel is instilled less frequently than balanced salt solution [8]. Instillation of 1.4 % sodium hyaluronate can also assist in making the corneal surface refractively consistent prior to commencing surgery; this procedure is preferred by the author.

Corneal Stromal Disease

Preoperative Considerations

Corneal stromal diseases, including corneal dystrophy and stromal scarring due to trauma, infectious or inflammatory conditions, can limit optical biometry measurements. For example, these diseases may impede the incident rays for laser interferometry, reducing the ability of partial coherence laser interferometry to measure the axial length of the eye. Conventional ultrasound biometry may therefore be used to measure the axial length of eyes with mild corneal opacity. However, noncontact optical biometry is less dependent on operators, providing more reliable and consistent results [9]. Another major concern arising in patients with corneal stromal diseases is the appropriateness of implanting advanced technology intraocular lenses (IOLs), including toric and multifocal IOLs. Toric IOLs in patients with stable keratoconus and forme fruste keratoconus, with less impaired spectacle-corrected vision, may reduce residual astigmatism, despite regular astigmatism being an absolute indication for toric IOLs. Implantation of advanced technology IOLs into patients who depend on rigid gas permeable contact lenses for vision correction seems inappropriate, because these IOLs produce additional internal astigmatism that cannot be corrected by contact lenses. Interestingly,

advanced technology IOLs have been reported to be beneficial in diseases such as keratoconus and irregular astigmatism due to previous surgical wounds or corneal opacity, conditions usually regarded as a contraindication to implantation (Fig. 16.1) [10, 11]. Additional evidence about the benefits and effectiveness of these IOLs may broaden surgical options in patients with corneal stromal diseases.

Intraoperative Considerations

Most corneal stromal diseases reduce the clarity of the cornea, which may significantly compromise the surgeon's view during cataract surgery. The surgical field may be optimized in some patients with localized corneal opacity by better positioning of the patient's head or eye, or increasing the magnification and modifying the intensity or direction of illumination. Most surgical steps may be completed through the limited area of the unaffected cornea (Fig. 16.2). However, these maneuvers may be insufficient for eyes with more diffuse or significant opacity. For example, usual coaxial illumination by a surgical microscope may result in backscattering and reflections from opaque cornea. Among the illumination techniques that can be employed to improve the intraoperative view are chandelier illumination and an endoilluminator from either outside or inside the eye [12, 13]. Capsular staining during capsulorhexis may also increase the surgical view. Although concerns have been raised about their potential toxicity [14], 0.1 % trypan blue and 0.125–0.5 % indocyanine green are frequently utilized in clinical practice [15, 16]. These vital dyes may also have stiffening effects on the lens capsule, increasing the possibility of completing capsulorhexis, even under situations involving limited surgical manipulation [17].

An adequately sized capsulorhexis is of the utmost importance throughout surgery in patients with a corneal comorbidity. If central opacity is large, a small sized capsulorhexis

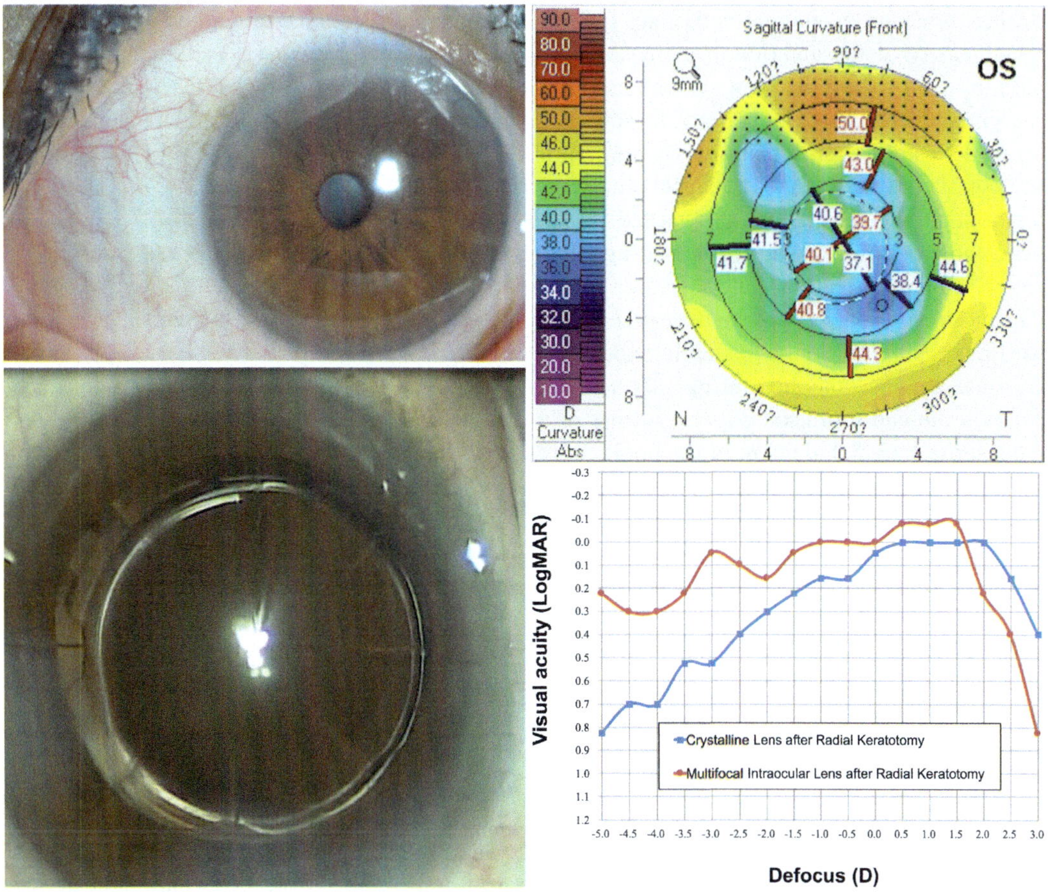

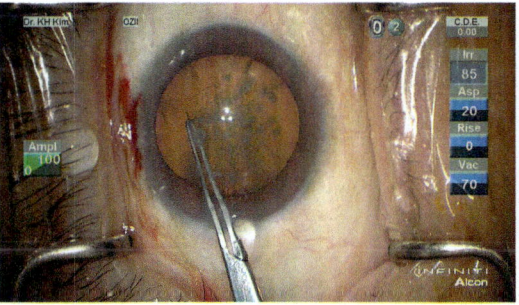
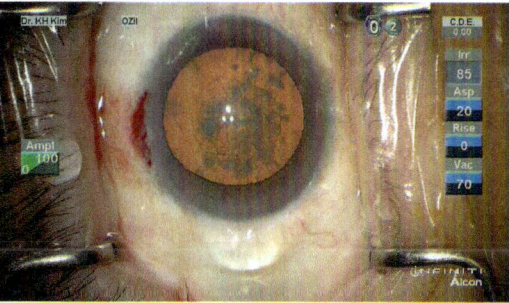

Fig. 16.1 Implantation of multifocal intraocular lens (IOL) significantly improved difficulty viewing near objects bilaterally in a 55-year-old woman with hyperopia who underwent bilateral radial keratotomy (RK) 18 years before. (*Top Left*) Slit-lamp examination showed 8 well-healed RK scars in each eye, with no visually significant lens opacities. (*Top Right*) Corneal topography using Pentacam revealed central flattening with irregularity in the left eye. (*Bottom Left*) 3 months after unilateral surgery using multifocal IOL, (*Bottom Right*) binocular uncorrected distant and near visual acuity improved to 20/20 and J1 from 20/25 and J9 or J10, respectively. Patient did not report any significant photic phenomena, and was satisfied with the results of treatment

Fig. 16.2 (*Left*) Corneal stromal diseases reduce the clarity of the cornea, which may significantly compromise the surgeon's view during cataract surgery. However, surgical steps may be started through the limited area of the unaffected cornea, and (*Right*) completed safely with optimizing the surgical field by better positioning of the patient's head or eye, or increasing the magnification and modifying the intensity or direction of illumination

during the stage of nucleofractis may imperil the integrity of the anterior or posterior capsule, by obstructing the views of the capsular margin and area of manipulation. In addition, an inadequately sized capsulorhexis may limit the use of conversion for extracapsular cataract extraction, as conversion is regarded as an acceptable option in complicated settings during phacoemulsification. Furthermore, if the capsulorhexis margin is located further inside the dilated pupil, the hook to stabilize the loose capsular-zonular complex during surgery may drag on the capsulorhexis edge, resulting in a capsular tear or dislodgment of the hook.

Severe diffuse opacity precludes starting capsulorhexis, which is regarded as a prerequisite for safe extracapsular cataract extraction. In this setting, simultaneous or staged keratoplasty should be considered along with cataract surgery. As long as a healthy endothelium can be ensured, deep anterior lamellar keratoplasty (DALK, the author's preference) can be performed. This method has several advantages, including the ability to undergo cataract surgery in a closed system, fewer postoperative refractive errors, increased wound strength due to an intact Descemet's membrane, and a reduced risk of graft rejection over the penetrating keratoplasty (PKP) (Fig. 16.3). Compared with simultaneous surgery [18, 19], staged keratoplasty (the author's preference), followed by cataract surgery, allows residual refractive errors to be corrected after keratoplasty. This can improve final visual outcomes, despites prolonged visual rehabilitation and a low but definite risk of endothelial cell loss after PKP [20]. The risk of endothelial cell loss during phacoemulsification after PKP may be reduced by using a soft-shell technique. In this method, the endothelium is protected by coating with a lower viscosity dispersive agent in addition to coating with the higher viscosity cohesive agent for surgical maneuvers [21]. For simultaneous surgery using the DALK technique [18, 19], the fluidics setting is adjusted to a low vacuum and flow rates, minimizing trauma to Descemet's membrane during

phacoemulsification after removal of the anterior stroma. Placing a high-viscosity ophthalmic viscosurgical device (OVD) over Descemet's membrane is also useful during simultaneous DALK (Fig. 16.4).

Corneal Endothelial Disease

Preoperative Considerations

As any surgical procedure may have a detrimental effect on endothelial cells, particular attention should be paid to cataract patients with corneal endothelial diseases. Corneal endothelial cell damage after cataract surgery was reported to be slight in eyes with a low endothelial cell density (ECD), comparable to that in eyes with a normal cell density [22]. However, preoperatively unhealthy endothelium may be jeopardized after surgery because of a low reservoir to compensate for impairment of the corneal endothelium, as shown by a study evaluating the effect of earlier cataract surgery in one eye on the progression to corneal decompensation in patients treated with bilateral PKP due to Fuchs' dystrophy [23]. A low ECD may indicate diseases such as corneal opacity, most likely due to viral or syphilitic keratitis; corneal guttata; Fuchs' dystrophy; endothelial injury from previous inflammation, surgery, or trauma; history of primary angle closure glaucoma attack or laser iridotomy; or pseudoexfoliation syndrome [22]. Therefore, careful preoperative evaluation of patients is necessary to identify those with corneal endothelial disease, followed by appropriate surgical planning. In patients undergoing staged operations, with keratoplasty planned after cataract extraction, possible refractive changes after keratoplasty should be considered when calculating IOL power for cataract surgery. Descemet stripping automated endothelial keratoplasty (DSAEK) has been reported to induce an average hyperopia of 1.1 D (range, 0.7 D–1.5 D) [24], because the shape of the graft, a diverging lens with a thin center and thick

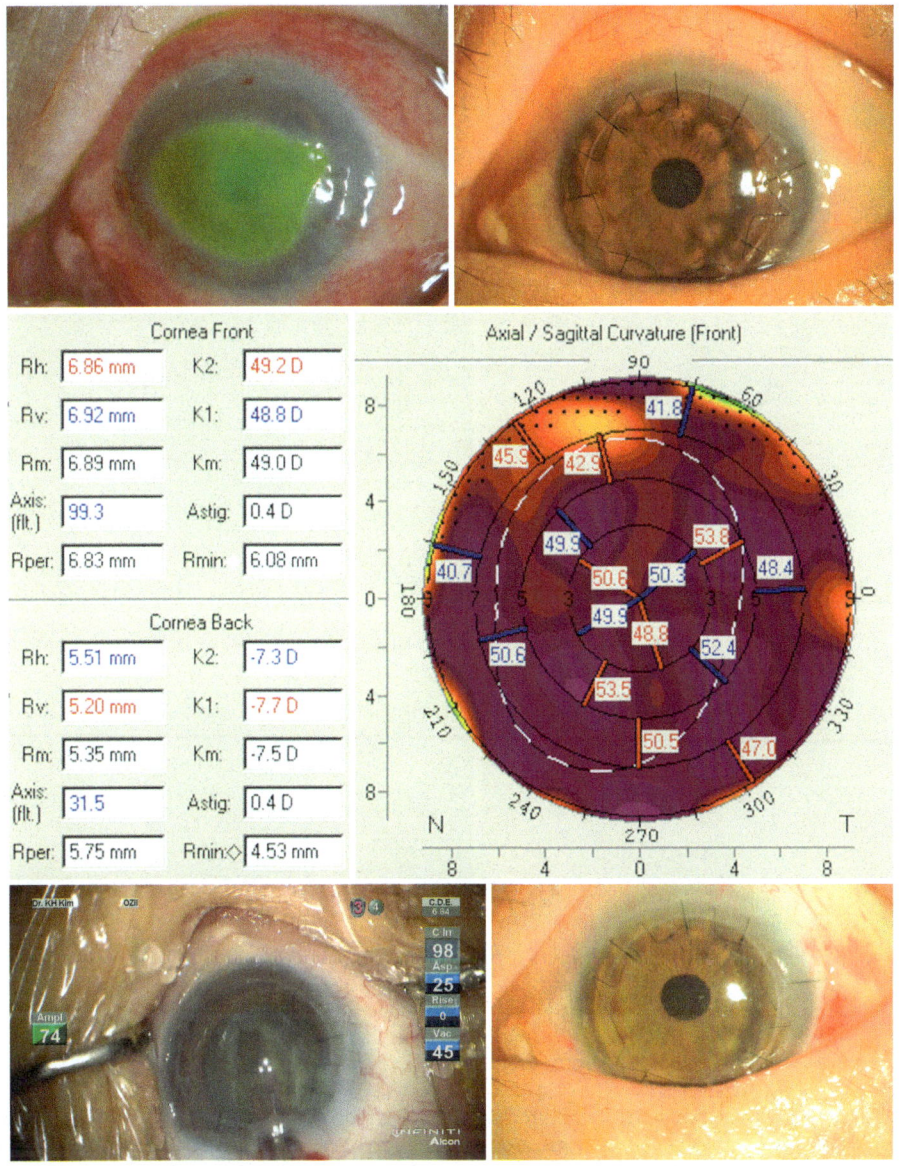

Fig. 16.3 A 67 year-old man with decreased vision of counting fingers, which could not be corrected by glasses, for 6 months was referred to my clinic. His medical history revealed that he had suffered from Trachoma since 40–50 years before and phototherapeutic keratectomy using excimer laser was performed 2 months prior to being referred. He also reported history of diabetes mellitus for 20 years. (*Top Left*) Slitlamp examination revealed pervasive epithelial defect, which was surrounded by the rim of hazy and loose epithelium, and stromal lysis. (*Top Right*) Under the diagnosis of neurotrophic keratopathy, deep anterior lamellar keratectomy was performed for both restoration of structural intergrity and visual rehabilitation. His uncorrected vision was improved to 20/80 1 month postoperatively and visually significant cataract was found through the clear cornea during slitlamp examination. (*Center Left* and *Right*) Corneal topography 1 month after keratoplasty showed clinically insignificant astigmatism, (*Bottom Left*) therefore phacoemulsification and intraocular lens implantation was performed. (*Bottom Right*) His uncorrected vision was improved to 20/25 3 months after cataract surgery and it has remained stable until the recent follow-up of 19 months after the surgery

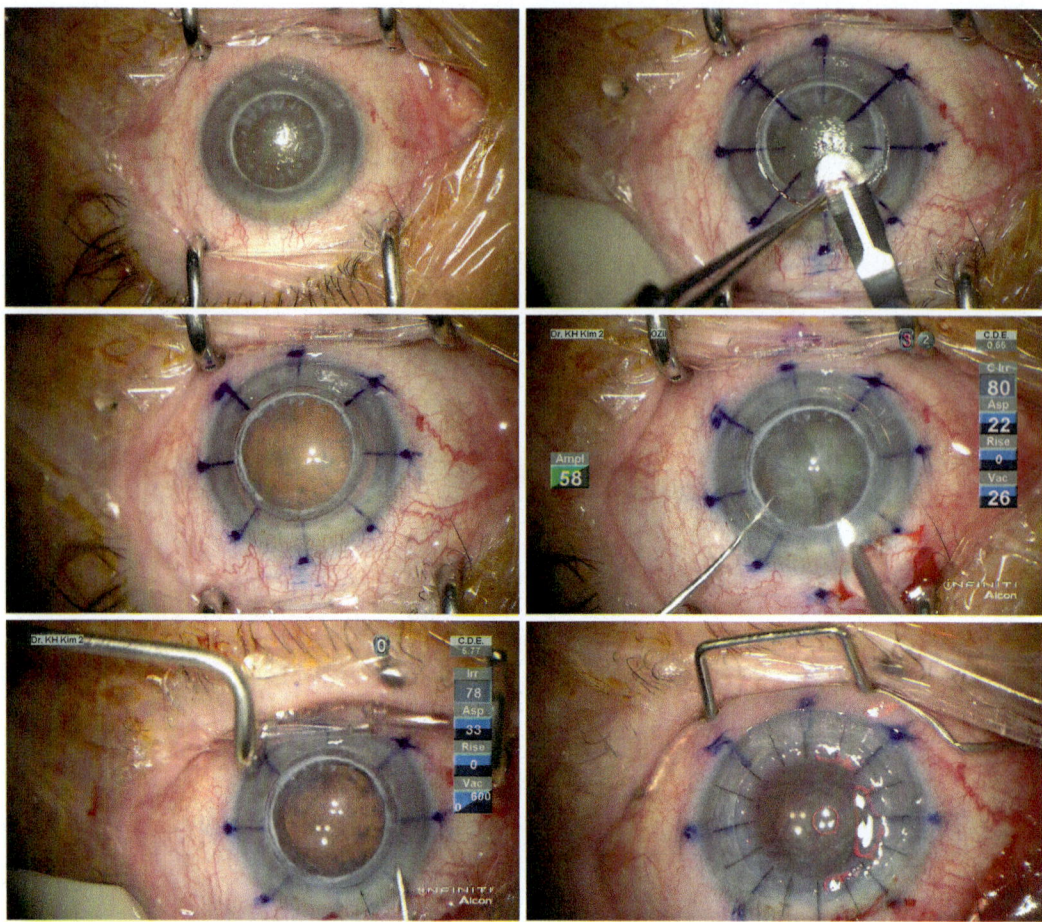

Fig. 16.4 A 78 year-old man was referred to my clinic for the treatment of recurred corneal dystrophy and cataract after penetrating keratoplasty. His medical history revealed that he underwent phototherapeutic keratectomy 2 years ago on the recurred Avellino dystrophy 10 years after penetrating keratoplasty, which was performed after the failure of previous phototherapeutic keratectomy 3 years earlier. Uncorrected distant vision of the diseased eye was 20/200 and it was not corrected by the glasses. Severe nuclear sclerosis was identified through slitlamp examination and cataract surgery with simultaneous keratoplasty was planned. (*Top Left*) Diffuse stromal opacity due to the corneal dystrophy significantly compromised surgical view. (*Top Right*) Through the lamellar keratec-tomy using a crescent knife, half thickness of the cornea was removed, (*Center Left*) thus surgical view was significantly improved. (*Center Right*) Frequent application of balanced salt solution or instillation of 1.4 % sodium hyaluronate assisted in making the corneal surface refractively consistent enough to perform procedures of phacoemulsification with no difficulty, (*Bottom Left*) and cataract surgery was completed without any complication. (*Bottom Right*) The sequential keratoplasty was performed to remove the residual opacity and replace the removed stroma. Patient reported a high level of satisfaction with improved vision (uncorrected distant vision of 20/40 and corrected distant vision of 20/25) 1 month after this cataract surgery with simultaneous keratoplasty

periphery, could deform the posterior corneal curvature [25]. A rational target for the cataract surgery before DSAEK may therefore be a postoperative refraction of −0.5 to −1.5 D. Although cataract surgery after keratoplasty may result in more accurate postoperative refraction, the risk of graft dislocation or loss of endothelial cells should be considered prior to using this approach. In selecting IOLs, aspherical IOLs may be implanted into patients with the same indications as those undergoing uncomplicated cataract surgery, considering that spherical aberration was reported to be unaffected by DSAEK [26]. If PKP is planned after cataract extraction, refractive changes should be considered during IOL power calculations, because the most frequent manifestations of ametropia after penetrating keratoplasty are astigmatism and myopia [24]. The mean amount of myopic astigmatism after PKP has been reported to be −4.3 D, but may be higher [27]. In addition, a meta-analysis comparing PKP and DALK showed similar refractive errors for the two approaches [28]. An average of the post-transplant corneal power by the surgeon may be utilized for cataract surgery before or during PKP or DALK. However, as these measurements may result in inaccurate results in calculating IOL power, and as toric IOLs implanted during cataract surgery after PKP successfully reduced manifest refraction [29], sequential cataract surgery after keratoplasty may be advantageous (Fig. 16.5). Sequential surgery may provide an additional opportunity to improve visual outcomes, despite the potential risk of endothelial cell loss from the graft, a loss that can be minimized using several techniques.

Intraoperative Considerations

A soft-shell technique may minimize endothelial cell loss during cataract surgery in patients with an unhealthy endothelium or after previous keratoplasty. Fluidics should also be adjusted for low vacuum and flow rate, and care should be exercised through the use of low amounts of ultrasound energy, as these low amounts may be necessary to avoid trauma to the endothelium. For nucleofractis, there is no evidence that any technique minimizes endothelial cell loss [30, 31], although the phaco chop technique is generally believed to use less ultrasound energy.

These general principles can be modified in patients undergoing concurrent cataract surgery and keratoplasty. First, the main incision for the introduction of the phacoemulsification hand piece can be made in the scleral tunnel (the author's preference), because, during the DSAEK procedure, endothelial grafts can be more safely implanted through the scleral tunnel than through a clear corneal incision. If Descemet membrane endothelial keratoplasty (DMEK) is planned, the same clear corneal incision, 2.2–2.8 mm in length, could be used for endothelial graft insertion after wound enlargement. The size and location of the graft in sequential endothelial keratoplasty should be considered when making corneal incisions for the secondary instruments. As the vertical meridian of the cornea is generally the shortest, a paracentesis wound with a longer tunnel located at 6 or 12 o'clock can be fully covered by the endothelial graft, blocking injection of air into the anterior chamber for the tamponade during keratoplasty. However, manipulation of instruments through paracentesis could enlarge the wound, making it difficult to maintain a stable anterior chamber with air tamponade due to air leakage. Therefore, designing the paracentesis wound so that it is slightly overlapped by the graft after air injection may minimize difficulties while attaching the donor graft (the author's preference).

If concurrent endothelial keratoplasty is planned, surgical views obscured by severe corneal edema may be improved by removing Descemet's membrane and the endothelium complex. Several capsular staining agents may also enhance the surgical view during the capsulorhexis stage. However, a dispersive type of OVD should be avoided when planning concurrent endothelial keratoplasty, because its remnants between the donor cornea and endothelial graft may disturb their appropriate attachment and risk graft dislocation after DSAEK. Furthermore, there is insufficient need to protect the endothelium during DSAEK to justify the use of dispersive OVD, despite its general use for endothelial protection. A cohesive type of OVD may be used, but should be removed completely after cataract surgery and its removal confirmed before endothelial keratoplasty.

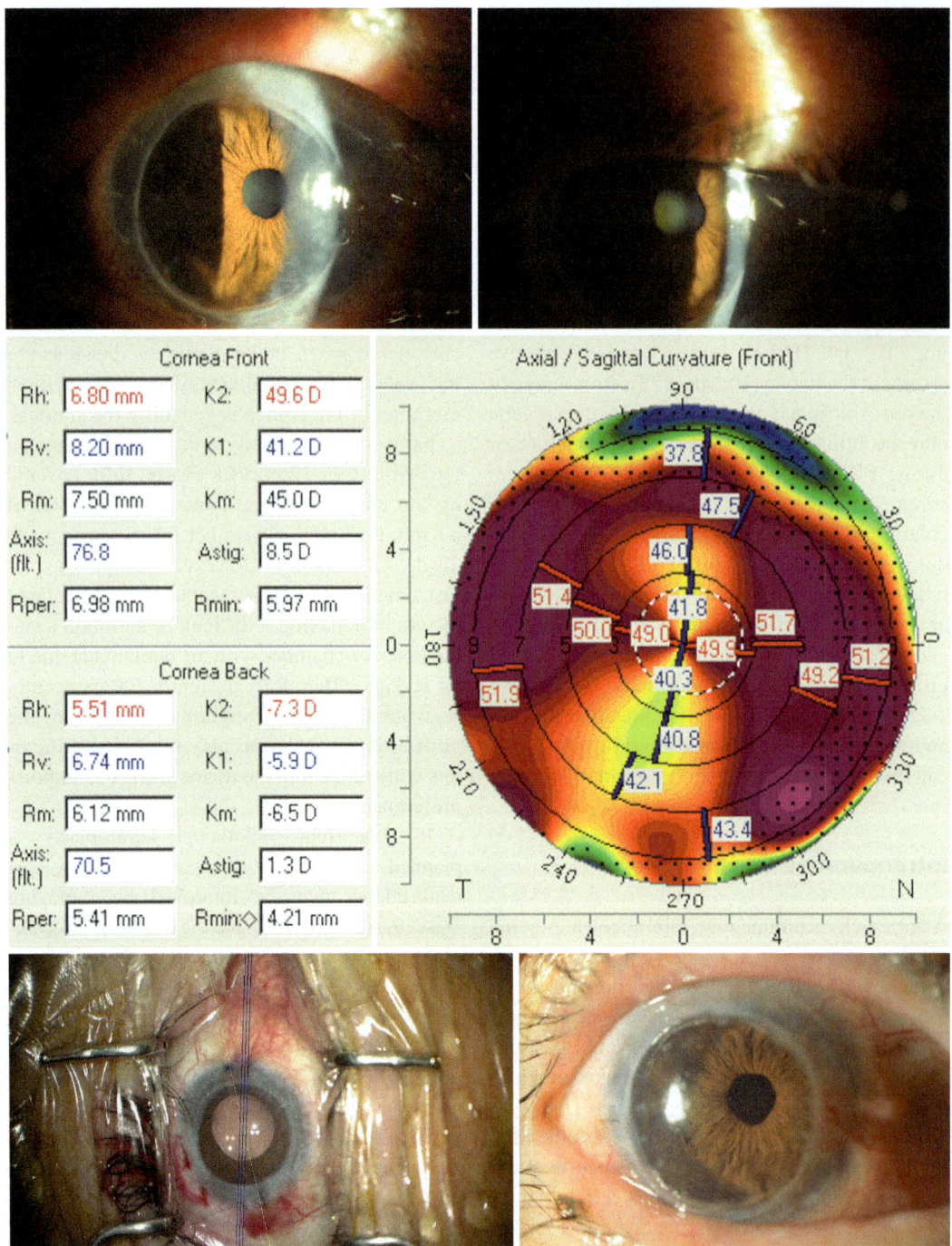

Fig. 16.5 A 68 year-old man with decreased vision was referred to my clinic. His uncorrected vision was checked as 20/200 and vision could not be corrected by glasses. His medical history revealed that he had underwent the penetrating keratoplasty due to corneal opacity 3 years before. (*Top Left* and *Right*) Slitlamp examination revealed that the corneal graft was relatively clear, but there was a significant cataract of nuclear sclerosis type. (*Center Left* and *Right*) Corneal topography showed severe astigmatism over 8 diopters, (*Bottom Left*) therefore toric intraocular lens implantation (Model 565 Precizon Toric; Ophtec BV, Groningen, Netherlands) was performed. (*Bottom Right*) Postoperative refraction at a follow up visit 3 months after the surgery was −0.25 −0.50 × 150 and his uncorrected vision was improved to 20/25

References

1. Greene JB, Mian SI. Cataract surgery in patients with corneal disease. Curr Opin Ophthalmol. 2013;24:9–14.
2. Kim P, Plugfelder S, Slomovic AR. Top 5 pearls to consider when implanting advanced-technology IOLs in patients with ocular surface disease. Int Ophthalmol Clin. 2012;52:51–8.
3. Movahedan A, Djalilian AR. Cataract surgery in the face of ocular surface disease. Curr Opin Ophthalmol. 2012;23:68–72.
4. Penn EA, Soong HK. Cataract surgery in allogeneic bone marrow transplant recipients with graft-versus-host disease(1). J Cataract Refract Surg. 2002;28:417–20.
5. Geerling G, Dart JK. Management and outcome of cataract surgery in ocular cicatricial pemphigoid. Graefe's Archive Clin Exp Ophthalmol = Albrecht von Graefes Archiv fur klinische und experimentelle Ophthalmologie. 2000;238:112–8.
6. Sangwan VS, Burman S. Cataract surgery in Stevens-Johnson syndrome. J Cataract Refract Surg. 2005;31:860–2.
7. Perez VL, Azar DT, Foster CS. Sterile corneal melting and necrotizing scleritis after cataract surgery in patients with rheumatoid arthritis and collagen vascular disease. Semin Ophthalmol. 2002;17:124–30.
8. Chen YA, Hirnschall N, Findl O. Comparison of corneal wetting properties of viscous eye lubricant and balanced salt solution to maintain optical clarity during cataract surgery. J Cataract Refract Surg. 2011;37:1806–8.
9. Findl O, Kriechbaum K, Sacu S, et al. Influence of operator experience on the performance of ultrasound biometry compared to optical biometry before cataract surgery. J Cataract Refract Surg. 2003;29:1950–5.
10. Kim KH, Seok KW, Kim WS. Multifocal intraocular lens results in correcting presbyopia in eyes after radial keratotomy. Eye Contact Lens. 2015. Epub ahead of print. PMID: 26625851. doi: 10.1097/ICL.0000000000000208.
11. Montano M, Lopez-Dorantes KP, Ramirez-Miranda A, Graue-Hernandez EO, Navas A. Multifocal toric intraocular lens implantation for forme fruste and stable keratoconus. J Refract Surg (Thorofare, NJ: 1995). 2014;30:282–5.
12. Nishimura A, Kobayashi A, et al. Endoillumination-assisted cataract surgery in a patient with corneal opacity. J Cataract Refract Surg. 2003;29:2277–80.
13. Oshima Y, Shima C, Maeda N, Tano Y. Chandelier retroillumination-assisted torsional oscillation for cataract surgery in patients with severe corneal opacity. J Cataract Refract Surg. 2007;33:2018–22.
14. Jacobs DS, Cox TA, Wagoner MD, Ariyasu RG, Karp CL. Capsule staining as an adjunct to cataract surgery: a report from the American Academy of Ophthalmology. Ophthalmology. 2006;113:707–13.
15. Melles GR, de Waard PW, Pameyer JH, Beekhuis Houdijn W. Trypan blue capsule staining to visualize the capsulorhexis in cataract surgery. J Cataract Refract Surg. 1999;25:7–9.
16. Rodrigues EB, Costa EF, Penha FM, et al. The use of vital dyes in ocular surgery. Surv Ophthalmol. 2009;54:576–617.
17. Haritoglou C, Mauell S, Schumann RG, et al. Increase in lens capsule stiffness caused by vital dyes. J Cataract Refract Surg. 2013;39:1749–52.
18. Muraine MC, Collet A, Brasseur G. Deep lamellar keratoplasty combined with cataract surgery. Arch Ophthalmol (Chicago, Ill : 1960) 2002;120:812–5.
19. Panda A, Sethi HS, Jain M, Nindra Krishna S, Gupta AK. Deep anterior lamellar keratoplasty with phacoemulsification. J Cataract Refract Surg. 2011;37:122–6.
20. Nagra PK, Rapuano CJ, Laibson PL, Kunimoto DY, Kay M, Cohen EJ. Cataract extraction following penetrating keratoplasty. Cornea. 2004;23:377–9.
21. Arshinoff SA. Dispersive-cohesive viscoelastic soft shell technique. J Cataract Refract Surg. 1999;25:167–73.
22. Hayashi K, Yoshida M, Manabe S, Hirata A. Cataract surgery in eyes with low corneal endothelial cell density. J Cataract Refract Surg. 2011;37:1419–25.
23. Afshari NA, Pittard AB, Siddiqui A, Klintworth GK. Clinical study of Fuchs corneal endothelial dystrophy leading to penetrating keratoplasty: a 30-year experience. Arch Ophthalmol (Chicago, Ill : 1960) 2006;124:777–80.
24. Lee WB, Jacobs DS, Musch DC, Kaufman SC, Reinhart WJ, Shtein RM. Descemet's stripping endothelial keratoplasty: safety and outcomes: a report by the American Academy of Ophthalmology. Ophthalmology. 2009;116:1818–30.
25. Scorcia V, Matteoni S, Scorcia GB, Scorcia G, Busin M. Pentacam assessment of posterior lamellar grafts to explain hyperopization after Descemet's stripping automated endothelial keratoplasty. Ophthalmology. 2009;116:1651–5.
26. Clemmensen K, Ivarsen A, Hjortdal J. Changes in corneal power after descemet stripping automated endothelial keratoplasty. J Refract Surg (Thorofare, NJ : 1995) 2015;31:807–12.
27. Claesson M, Armitage WJ, Fagerholm P, Stenevi U. Visual outcome in corneal grafts: a preliminary analysis of the Swedish Corneal Transplant Register. Br J Ophthalmol. 2002;86:174–80.
28. Chen G, Tzekov R, Li W, Jiang F, Mao S, Tong Y. Deep anterior lamellar keratoplasty versus penetrating keratoplasty: a meta-analysis of randomized controlled trials. Cornea. 2016;35:169–74.
29. Wade M, Steinert RF, Garg S, Farid M, Gaster R. Results of toric intraocular lenses for post-penetrating keratoplasty astigmatism. Ophthalmology. 2014;121:771–7.
30. Park JH, Lee SM, Kwon JW, et al. Ultrasound energy in phacoemulsification: a comparative analysis of phaco-chop and stop-and-chop techniques according to the degree of nuclear density. Ophthalmic Surg Lasers Imaging: Off J Int Soc Imaging Eye. 2010;41:236–41.
31. Storr-Paulsen A, Norregaard JC, Ahmed S, Storr-Paulsen T, Pedersen TH. Endothelial cell damage after cataract surgery: divide-and-conquer versus phaco-chop technique. J Cataract Refract Surg. 2008;34:996–1000.

Improvements in instrumentation and surgical techniques have enhanced patient expectations for surgical outcomes. Presbyopia, which results from a loss of accommodation, is considered the main reason for dissatisfaction after conventional cataract surgery, and remains a significant challenge for ophthalmologists.

Corrective techniques for presbyopia include spectacle correction, monovision using corrective lenses or surgery, multifocal corneal excimer laser ablation, and refractive lens exchange with either multifocal or accommodating intraocular lenses (IOLs) [1]. Recently introduced presbyopia-correcting IOLs may enhance patient satisfaction. These IOLs have two or more focal points, thus extending their range of vision. In contrast, conventional monofocal IOLs have a single fixed focal length. Multifocal IOLs, however, have various adverse effects, including reduced contrast sensitivity and subjective experiences of glare and halo [2]. Furthermore, not every currently available IOL is suitable for every patient, due to the complexity of lifestyle choices and personality dynamics or the inherent anatomy and physiology of the eye [3].

Preoperative Considerations

A small amount of astigmatism does not degrade visual acuity in normal eyes [4], and the visual benefits of precise correction of astigmatism < 0.5 D are limited. In contrast, control of astigmatism is of critical importance for satisfactory results of multifocal IOL implantation after cataract surgery, as astigmatism was the greatest cause of patient dissatisfaction after multifocal IOL implantation [5]. The presence of astigmatism in eyes with a diffractive multifocal IOL compromised visual acuities at distance, emphasizing the importance of controlling astigmatism [6]. In that study, the corrected distance visual acuity and distance corrected intermediate visual acuity at 0.5 m in eyes with astigmatism of 1.50 D and 2.00 D were significantly worse following multifocal than monofocal IOL implantation, although the distance corrected near visual acuity was similar in the two groups [6]. Therefore, careful preoperative evaluation of astigmatism is necessary for relevant surgical planning. Corneal topography may provide useful information about corneal astigmatism, such as regularity, tear film quality, aberration, and posterior astigmatism. Age-related changes in astigmatism have been found to differ on the anterior and posterior corneal surfaces, as measured by conventional keratometry on the anterior surface and by a specific instrument such as a Scheimpflug analyzer and anterior segment optical coherence tomography on the posterior corneal surface [7, 8]. An IOL power calculation using only a measure of anterior corneal keratometric may not select the ideal power, increasing the risk of patient dissatisfaction with this procedure. Because a vertically steep posterior corneal curvature resulted in against-the-rule astigmatism, calculations using only the anterior corneal keratometric value may result in an overestimation of total corneal astigmatism in eyes with with-the-rule anterior corneal astigmatism or an underestimation in eyes with against-the-rule anterior corneal astigmatism. Preoperative evaluation of the macula and identification of retinal comorbidities are also important for favorable outcomes after cataract surgery using presbyopia-correcting IOLs.

Careful patient selection through preoperative evaluation and counselling are also important, especially for multifocal IOLs. Pupil size may affect the performance of multifocal IOLs and visual outcomes. For example, the Strehl ratio of IOLs was found to decrease in proportion to pupil size [9]. Near focusing did not occur in individuals with refractive IOL and pupils smaller than 3.5 mm, resulting in poor image quality. Nevertheless, the image quality of refractive IOLs was superior to that of diffractive-refractive IOLs at distance and with small pupils. Therefore the selection of IOL type should consider the pupil size of each eye. Angle kappa, the angle resulting from the misalignment between the pupillary axis and the visual axis, should also be considered preoperatively when planning implantation of multifocal IOLs. In eyes with a small angle kappa, the incident ray could pass through the central area of the multifocal IOL. However, in eyes with larger angle kappa, the incident ray may pass through the edge of the ring of the refractive multifocal IOL and be scattered, resulting in photic phenomena [10]. In addition, the angle kappa at which the incident ray passes through the first ring's edge area of diffractive multifocal IOLs is affected by corneal power, effective lens position, and axial length [11]. Therefore, implantation of diffractive multifocal IOLs into eyes with a large angle kappa and a shallow anterior chamber depth may be a risk factor for pronounced photic phenomena, suggesting the use of multifocal IOLs not having a diffractive design. Due to these complex etiologies, photic phenomena were reported to be the main presenting symptoms in dissatisfied patients who underwent cataract surgery using multifocal IOLs [5]. Moreover, a systematic review comparing visual outcomes in patients implanted with multifocal and monofocal IOLs showed that the rate of these adverse visual phenomena was significantly higher in patients implanted with multifocal IOLs [2]. Because enthusiasm for spectacle independence and patient characteristics may be related to the gratification experienced by a patient following multifocal IOL implantation, patients planning multifocal IOL implantation should be counseled about the possible adverse effects, as well as about the relative advantages and disadvantages of improved near vision and spectacle independence. Visual life activities should also be considered in patients planning to undergo implantation of multifocal IOLs. Conventional multifocal IOLs have two focal points, resulting in distinctive defocus curve profiles, with two peaks of optimum visual acuity, one at distance and the other at near. Because working distance and visual outcome at near vary according to the additional power for near vision, preoperative counseling may also help in selecting the additional power of multifocal IOLs. Perfect multifocal IOLs have not yet been introduced, although the gap between the real and ideal is narrowing. Recently introduced low-additional-power multifocal IOLs may provide better intermediate and even near vision without significantly reducing distant vision or compromising contrast sensitivity or ocular optical quality. These new lenses may optimize overall patient satisfaction by reducing visual disturbances and spectacle needs for daily life activities (Fig. 17.1 and Table 17.1) [12].

Since the introduction of excimer laser technology, many patients have undergone refractive surgical procedures. As these patients have aged, the number undergoing cataract surgery who also underwent previous refractive surgery has increased markedly. Multifocal IOLs are rarely implanted after refractive surgery because of concerns about the reduction in image contrast associated with having two or more simultaneous focal points in order to extend range of vision, which may decrease further in proportion to the degree of corneal aberration, such as coma, spherical aberration, or first-order astigmatism,

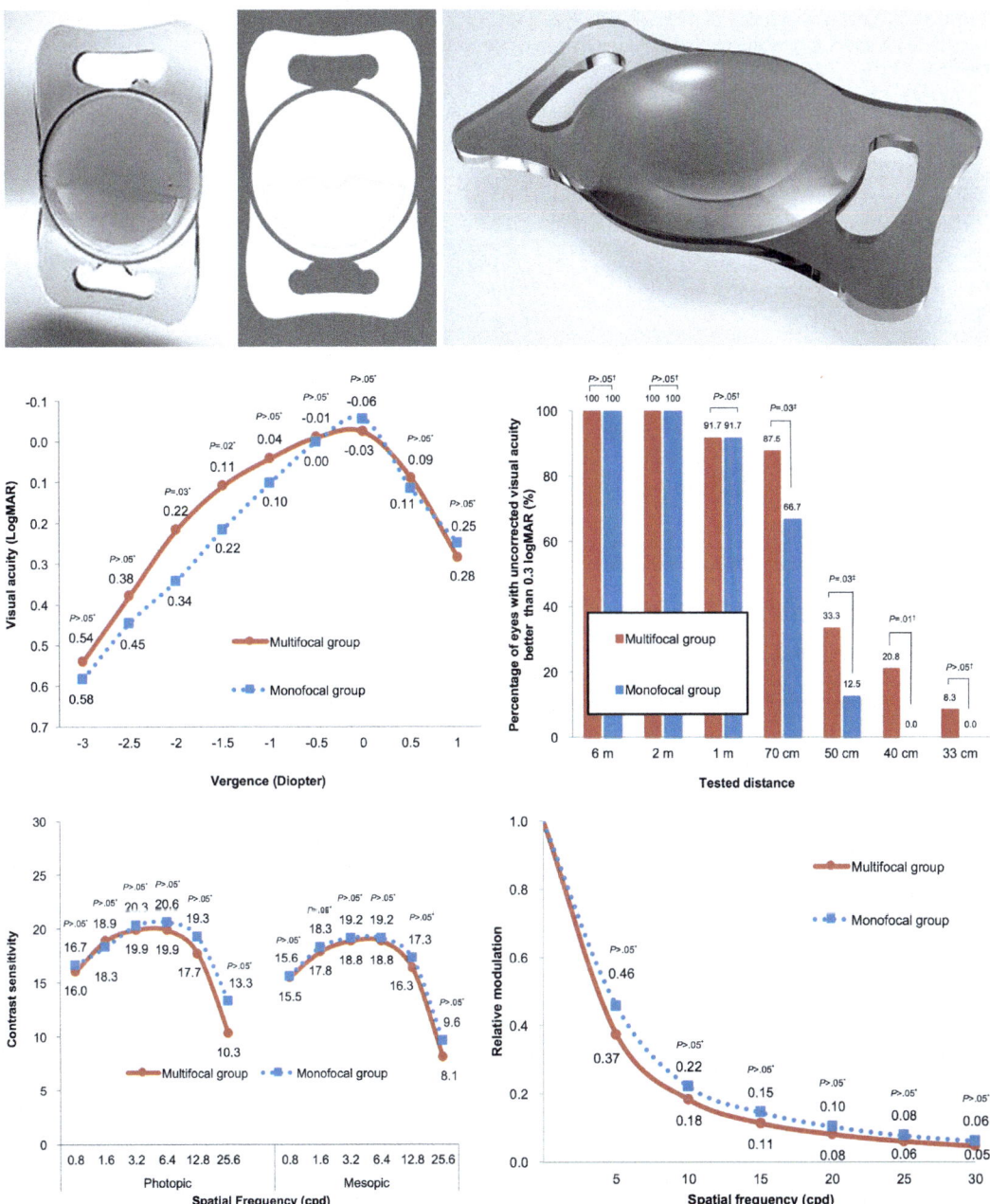

Fig. 17.1 Low-power-added multifocal IOLs (*Top Left*; LS313MF15, Oculentis, Germany) yielded better intermediate and near vision without increasing optical phenomena compared with monofocal IOLs (*Top Right*; CTS204, Carl Zeiss Meditec AG, Germany; unpublished data). (*Center Left*) Mean defocus curves following implantation of low-additional-power multifocal IOLs and conventional monofocal IOLs. Visual acuity at vergences of −1.5 and −2.0 D, equivalent to 66.7 cm and 50 cm, respectively, from the eye differed significantly in the two groups. (*Center Right*) Percentage of eyes with the logarithm of the minimal angle of resolution (log-

MAR) 0.3 or better. The percentage of eyes with vision better than 0.3 logMAR was significantly higher in the multifocal than in the monofocal group at 70 cm, 50 cm, and 40 cm. (*Bottom Left*) Mean contrast sensitivity function under photopic and scotopic conditions. Photopic and mesopic distance contrast sensitivities in the two groups did not differ significantly at any tested spatial frequency. (*Bottom Right*) Modulation transfer function in the two groups. There was no significant between-group difference in modulation transfer functions at all tested cycles per degree (cpds). *cpd* cycles per degree; * Mann–Whitney *U* test; † Fisher's exact test; ‡ Chi-squared test

Table 17.1 Low-power-added multifocal IOLs (LS313MF15, Oculentis, Germany) yielded better intermediate and near vision without increasing optical phenomena compared with monofocal IOLs (CTS204, Carl Zeiss Meditec AG, Germany [12])

Item[a]	Multifocal group (N=24)	Monofocal group (N=24)	P value
Visual disturbances (from 0 to 5)			
Glare	1.0±1.1	1.7±1.1	.21[b]
Color perception	0.3±0.7	0.1±0.3	.68[b]
Depth perception	0.1±0.2	0.3±0.6	.25[b]
Halos	1.3±1.6	0.8±0.9	.63[b]
Distorted vision	0.7±1.1	0.4±0.9	.35[b]
Blurred vision	1.4±1.5	0.8±1.1	.11[b]
Diplopia	0.3±0.7	0.6±1.1	.68[b]
Visual lifestyle activities (from 0 to 5)			
Watching television or movie	0.4±0.6	0.9±1.0	.32[b]
Working outside or playing sports	0.4±1.0	0.6±0.9	.39[b]
Reading/near work	2.2±1.6	2.6±1.4	.63[b]
Computer/cooking/shopping	0.5±0.7	1.5±0.5	.03[b]
Using a cell phone/shaving/applying make up	1.1±1.3	1.3±1.5	.58[b]
Driving at night	1.0±1.1	1.6±1.1	.32[b]
Driving at rain	1.1±1.0	0.9±0.9	.72[b]
Spectacle use (from 0 to 3)			
For distance vision	0.4±1.0	1.3±1.4	.15[b]
For intermediate vision	1.0±1.4	2.0±0.9	.04[b]
For near vision	1.4±1.4	2.6±1.3	.08[b]
Overall satisfaction (from 0 to 10)			
	8.1±1.1	6.7±1.3	.02[b]

Postoperative scores for visual disturbances, lifestyle activities, spectacle use, and overall satisfaction, as determined by questionnaires following implantation of low-additional-power multifocal intraocular lenses and conventional monofocal intraocular lenses

[a]The response rating scales: visual disturbance and lifestyle activities, *0* no difficulty, *1* minimal difficulty, *2* and *3* moderate difficulty, *4* and *5* severe difficulty; spectacle use, *0* never, *1* rarely or occasionally, *2* often and *3* always; overall satisfaction, range from 0 (least satisfied) to 10 (most satisfied)

[b]Mann–Whitney *U* test

when implanting multifocal IOLs [3]. However, technological developments in the manufacture of IOLs have widened their application, even in patients who have previously undergone radial keratotomy [13]. Aberrations due to complex distortion of the cornea and the inability to predict refractive outcomes of cataract surgery in these patients have limited the implantation of multifocal IOLs [14, 15]. Specifically designed IOLs, with minimal interface and a limited zone producing different foci, may result in minimal aberration, thereby minimizing the aberrational effects produced by the deformed cornea after radial keratotomy.

Intraoperative Considerations

In an experimental study using an artificial model eye [16], the modulation transfer function (MTF) of refractive-diffractive IOLs was found to be more significantly affected by the decentration than the tilt of the IOL. Decentration of 0.2–0.4 mm reduced the cutoff frequency from 50 to 40 cycles per degree (cpd), but it was stable at all frequencies with a tilt of 2–5 degrees. Another study found that the effects on MTFs and near images are dependent on the design of multifocal IOLs, with clinically relevant effects not occurring at decentrations ≤ 0.75 mm. These findings together indicate that the favorable outcomes are highly dependent on the centration of multifocal IOL. A complete and well-centered continuous curvilinear capsulorhexis (CCC) is a prerequisite for good centration of an IOL. Another factor affecting the centration of an IOL is the presence of zonular weakness. Standard capsular tension rings (CTRs) may be useful in eyes with mild zonular instability, including those with small, localized zonular dialysis or mild diffuse zonular weakness [17]. Moreover, the combined use of a CTR and a multifocal IOL provided better predictability and increased the intraocular optical performance when compared with the multifocal IOL alone [18]. Because the IOL displacement attributable to capsular contraction is reduced when cataract surgery involves the posterior CCC [19], primary posterior CCC during cataract surgery using multifocal IOLs may stabilize the IOL and improve surgical outcomes.

The effect of anterior capsular tear on centration is unclear [20–22]. Although capsular fibrosis may not provide ideal stability of the IOL, it may provide sufficient stability. Implantation of multifocal IOLs into eyes with anterior capsular tears may therefore yield acceptable surgical results. Implantation of multifocal IOLs into eyes with posterior capsular tears is not categorically contraindicated, because a posterior capsular tear could be converted to a posterior CCC, as the stability of the IOL may increase after surgery due to capsular fibrosis and shrinkage [19]. The IOL can also be fixed through various types of optic capturing techniques, even in the absence of posterior capsular support [23, 24]. However, implantation of a single-piece IOL into the sulcus should be avoided because it carries risks of several complications, including pigment dispersion, iris transillumination defects, dysphotopsia, elevated intraocular pressure, intraocular hemorrhage, and cystoid macular edema (Fig. 17.2) [25].

Postoperative Considerations

Because contrast sensitivity is reduced as the range of vision is extended, it is generally recommended that multifocal IOLs should be implanted bilaterally rather than unilaterally. However, unilateral implantation into the dominant eye may yield satisfactory results, although bilateral implantation of refractive or diffractive multifocal IOLs provided better outcomes [26, 27]. A mix-and-match study found that spectacle independence and visual outcomes were similar following unilateral or bilateral implantation of diffractive and refractive multifocal IOLs [28]. Therefore, unilateral implantation can be considered an option for selected patients, including younger persons with monocular cataract. However, this option is not applicable to functionally one-eyed patients, because the lack of compensatory visual contribution of a second eye would result in failure to correct an unavoidable reduction in contrast sensitivity and would not achieve the level of uncorrected visual function resulting from bilateral implantation of multifocal IOLs [3]. Patients with strabismus with alternation of fixation eye, or alternating monofixator, would also not have a summation benefit from simultaneous binocular multifocal vision. In practice, monofixation status may easily be missed, especially in patients with hyperopia and small-angle esotropia. Because these patients may also have mild amblyopia due to strabismus, the reduction in contrast sensitivity may be exacerbated. The performance of a four prism base-out test is highly recommended in patients with high hyperopia [3].

Despite careful preoperative evaluation and proper intraoperative techniques, some patients have reported dissatisfaction with the outcomes of multifocal IOL implantation [5, 29]. Reasons for dissatisfaction include blurred vision and photic phenomena, due primarily to residual refractive error, posterior capsular opacity, and/ or large pupil size. Relatively small amounts of refractive errors can be treated with spectacle correction or excimer laser. Laser in situ keratomileusis (LASIK) was found effective in treating patients with residual refractive errors of myopia (< -3.5 diopters (D)), hyperopia (< 1.25 D), and astigmatism (< 3.0 D) after multifocal IOL implantation [30]. Excimer laser including photorefractive keratectomy and LASIK may have advantages in avoiding risks of damage to intraocular structures, including

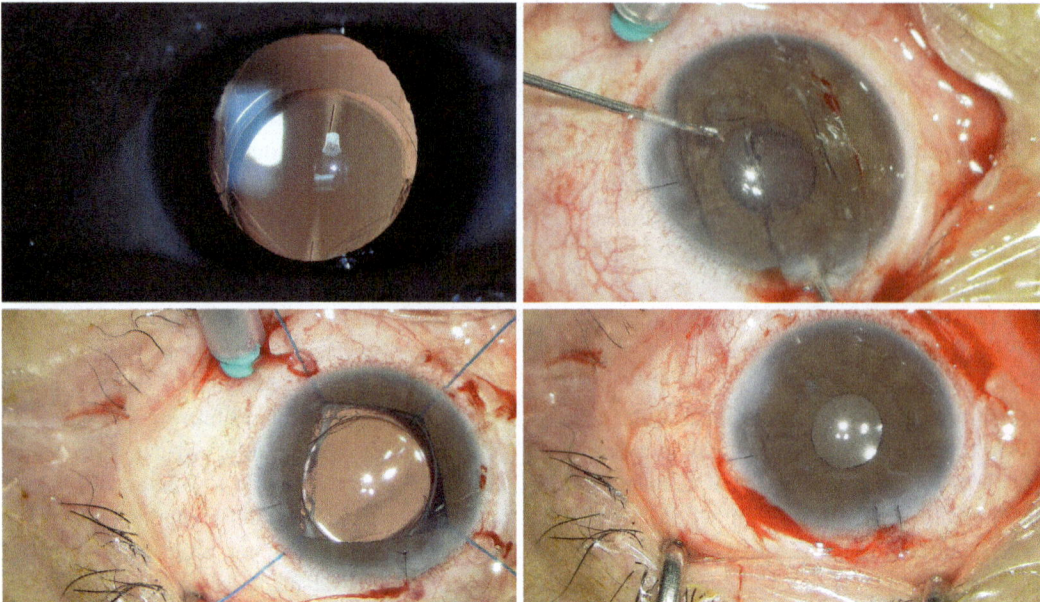

Fig. 17.2 A 54-year-old man with decreased and blurred vision was referred to my clinic after surgeries at other hospitals. His medical history revealed implantation of multifocal intraocular lens (IOL; LS313MF30, Oculentis, Germany) in the capsular bag in spite of posterior capsular rupture during primary cataract surgery 3 months prior, and the IOL dislocation into the vitreous cavity led to total vitrectomy and reposition of the dislocated IOL into the sulcus 1 month ago. (*Top Left*) Slitlamp examination showed multifocal IOL with a rotational asymmetric design was located in the sulcus and dislocated inferiorly. Considering the design of this IOL with overall length (11.0 mm) and thickness, and consequent complications such as a dislocation and a long-standing inflammation due to iris chafing, implanting this in the sulcus should be avoided. (*Top Right*) Due to a large posterior capsular opening and consequent lack of support in this case, infusion cannula was inserted at pars plana and pharmacologic miosis was induced during removal of the multifocal IOL. The characteristic design of this lens also may complicate removal procedures different from conventional IOLs. (*Bottom Left*) Monofocal multipiece IOL with haptics made of polymethylmethacrylate was implanted into the sulcus due to its tolerability to the decentration and appropriacy for the sulcus implantation. (*Bottom Right*) Centration of the IOL and any pupillary distortion were checked at the end of the surgery

the corneal endothelium. However, implantation of supplementary IOLs using a piggyback technique or IOL exchange can be considered for the correction of significant ametropia because the former was found to increase aberration in proportion to the ablation depth and to have detrimental effects on contrast sensitivity. Although posterior capsular opacity may cause photic phenomena, posterior capsulotomy using a neodymium: YAG (Nd: YAG) laser should be delayed until a causal relationship between posterior capsule opacification (PCO) and subjective symptoms of blurred vision or photic phenomena is confirmed, as the posterior capsular opening may complicate exchange of IOLs (Fig. 17.2). Blurred vision after implantation of refractive multifocal IOLs with rotational asym-

metry may be due to the intraocular orientation of the IOL. An experimental study showed that image quality varied significantly in accordance with changes in orientation of specific IOLs and that the mean differences in an image quality parameter (visually modulated transfer function metric) and modulation transfer function between the worst and best orientations of the IOL for distance vision were 58 % and 5 cpd, respectively [31]. Therefore, patients reporting unsatisfactory results following implantation of multifocal IOLs with rotational asymmetric design could be treated by rotating the IOL to its optimal orientation, which may differ among individuals. Large pupil size causing photic phenomena could be treated by instillation of brimonidine.

References

1. Kashani S, Mearza AA, Claoue C. Refractive lens exchange for presbyopia. Cont Lens Anterior Eye J British Cont Lens Ass. 2008;31:117–21.

2. Leyland M, Zinicola E. Multifocal versus monofocal intraocular lenses in cataract surgery: a systematic review. Ophthalmology. 2003;110:1789–98.

3. Braga-Mele R, Chang D, Dewey S, et al. Multifocal intraocular lenses: relative indications and contraindications for implantation. J Cataract Refract Surg. 2014;40:313–22.

4. Villegas EA, Alcon E, Artal P. Minimum amount of astigmatism that should be corrected. J Cataract Refract Surg. 2014;40:13–9.

5. de Vries NE, Webers CA, Touwslager WR, et al. Dissatisfaction after implantation of multifocal intraocular lenses. J Cataract Refract Surg. 2011;37:859–65.

6. Hayashi K, Manabe S, Yoshida M, Hayashi H. Effect of astigmatism on visual acuity in eyes with a diffractive multifocal intraocular lens. J Cataract Refract Surg. 2010;36:1323–9.

7. Koch DD, Ali SF, Weikert MP, Shirayama M, Jenkins R, Wang L. Contribution of posterior corneal astigmatism to total corneal astigmatism. J Cataract Refract Surg. 2012;38:2080–7.

8. Ueno Y, Hiraoka T, Beheregaray S, Miyazaki M, Ito M, Oshika T. Age-related changes in anterior, posterior, and total corneal astigmatism. J Refract Surg (Thorofare, NJ: 1995). 2014;30:192–7.

9. Artigas JM, Menezo JL, Peris C, Felipe A, Diaz-Llopis M. Image quality with multifocal intraocular lenses and the effect of pupil size: comparison of refractive and hybrid refractive-diffractive designs. J Cataract Refract Surg. 2007;33:2111–7.

10. Prakash G, Prakash DR, Agarwal A, Kumar DA, Agarwal A, Jacob S. Predictive factor and kappa angle analysis for visual satisfactions in patients with multifocal IOL implantation. Eye (Lond). 2011;25:1187–93.

11. Karhanova M, Pluhacek F, Mlcak P, Vlacil O, Sin M, Maresova K. The importance of angle kappa evaluation for implantation of diffractive multifocal intraocular lenses using pseudophakic eye model. Acta Ophthalmol. 2015;93:e123–8.

12. Kim KH, Kim WS. Visual outcome and patient satisfaction of low-power-added multifocal intraocular lens. Eye Contact Lens. 2016. Epub ahead of print. doi: 10.1097/ICL.0000000000000314.

13. Kim KH, Seok KW, Kim WS. Multifocal intraocular lens results in correcting presbyopia in eyes after radial keratotomy. Eye Contact Lens. 2015. Epub ahead of print. PMID: 26625851. doi: 10.1097/ICL.0000000000000208.

14. Demill DL, Hsu M, Moshirfar M. Evaluation of the American Society of Cataract and Refractive Surgery intraocular lens calculator for eyes with prior radial keratotomy. Clin Ophthalmol (Auckland, NZ). 2011;5:1243–7.

15. Chen L, Mannis MJ, Salz JJ, Garcia-Ferrer FJ, Ge J. Analysis of intraocular lens power calculation in post-radial keratotomy eyes. J Cataract Refract Surg. 2003;29:65–70.

16. Montes-Mico R, Lopez-Gil N, Perez-Vives C, Bonaque S, Ferrer-Blasco T. In vitro optical performance of nonrotational symmetric and refractive-diffractive aspheric multifocal intraocular lenses: impact of tilt and decentration. J Cataract Refract Surg. 2012;38:1657–63.

17. Hasanee K, Butler M, Ahmed II. Capsular tension rings and related devices: current concepts. Curr Opin Ophthalmol. 2006;17:31–41.

18. Alio JL, Elkady B, Ortiz D, Bernabeu G. Microincision multifocal intraocular lens with and without a capsular tension ring: optical quality and clinical outcomes. J Cataract Refract Surg. 2008;34:1468–75.

19. Kim KH, Kim WS. Intraocular lens stability and refractive outcomes after cataract surgery using primary posterior continuous curvilinear capsulorrhexis. Ophthalmology. 2010;117:2278–86.

20. Oner FH, Durak I, Soylev M, Ergin M. Long-term results of various anterior capsulotomies and radial tears on intraocular lens centration. Ophthalmic Surg Lasers. 2001;32:118–23.

21. Davison JA. Analysis of capsular bag defects and intraocular lens positions for consistent centration. J Cataract Refract Surg. 1986;12:124–9.

22. Haigh PM, Lloyd IC, Lavin MJ. Implantation of foldable intraocular lenses in the presence of anterior capsular tears. Eye (Lond). 1995;9(Pt 4):442–5.

23. Gimbel HV, DeBroff BM. Intraocular lens optic capture. J Cataract Refract Surg. 2004;30:200–6.

24. Jones JJ, Oetting TA, Rogers GM, Jin GJ. Reverse optic capture of the single-piece acrylic intraocular lens in eyes with posterior capsule rupture. Ophthalmic Surg Lasers Imaging Off J Int Soc Imaging Eye. 2012;43:480–8.

25. Chang DF, Masket S, Miller KM, et al. Complications of sulcus placement of single-piece acrylic intraocular lenses: recommendations for backup IOL implantation following posterior capsule rupture. J Cataract Refract Surg. 2009;35:1445–58.

26. Shoji N, Shimizu K. Binocular function of the patient with the refractive multifocal intraocular lens. J Cataract Refract Surg. 2002;28:1012–7.

27. Cionni RJ, Osher RH, Snyder ME, Nordlund ML. Visual outcome comparison of unilateral versus bilateral implantation of apodized diffractive multifocal intraocular lenses after cataract extraction: prospective 6-month study. J Cataract Refract Surg. 2009;35:1033–9.

28. Yoon SY, Song IS, Kim JY, Kim MJ, Tchah H. Bilateral mix-and-match versus unilateral multifocal intraocular lens implantation: long-term comparison. J Cataract Refract Surg. 2013;39:1682–90.

29. Woodward MA, Randleman JB, Stulting RD. Dissatisfaction after multifocal intraocular lens implantation. J Cataract Refract Surg. 2009;35:992–7.

30. Muftuoglu O, Prasher P, Chu C, et al. Laser in situ keratomileusis for residual refractive errors after apodized diffractive multifocal intraocular lens implantation. J Cataract Refract Surg. 2009;35:1063–71.

31. Bonaque-Gonzalez S, Rios S, Amigo A, Lopez-Gil N. Influence on visual quality of intraoperative orientation of asymmetric intraocular lenses. J Refract Surg (Thorofare, NJ: 1995). 2015;31:651–7.

The manufacturer's authorised representative in the EU is Springer
Nature Customer Service Centre GmbH, Europaplatz 3, 69115 Heidelberg,
Germany. If you have any concerns regarding our products, please
contact ProductSafety@springernature.com

Printed and bound by CPI Group (UK) Ltd, Croydon, CR0 4YY
23/04/2026
02095596-0005